Echocardiography Illust

Volume 4

Echocardiography Illustrated
Coronary Artery TERRITORIES

EchoPal™

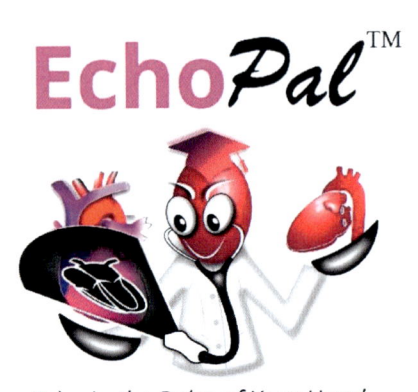

Echo in the Palm of Your Hand

Contact:
Author@EchoScope.org

Echo Stethoscope Academy Project

For printed Wall Charts and related Apps.
Kindle eBook edition @ Amazon.com

Echocardiography Illustrated
Coronary Artery TERRITORIES

Bernard E. Bulwer, MD, FASE
Founder and Project Director
Echo Stethoscope Academy Project
Longwood Medical and Academic Area
Boston, Massachusetts, USA

Noninvasive Cardiovascular Research
Cardiovascular Division, Brigham and Women's Hospital,
Harvard Medical School Teaching Affiliate
Boston, Massachusetts, USA

Formerly:
*Associate Professor and Program Director,
Diagnostic Medical Sonography-Echocardiography
School of Medical Imaging and Therapeutics
MCPHS University, Boston, Massachusetts, USA*

*Advanced Fellow in Noninvasive Cardiology-Echocardiography
Brigham and Women's Hospital, Harvard Medical School
Boston, Massachusetts, USA*

*Lown Fellow in Cardiovascular Disease
Lown Cardiovascular Center/Brigham and Women's Hospital,
Harvard Medical School, Boston, Massachusetts, USA*

*Director of Medical Services and the Cardiac Program
Karl Heusner Memorial Hospital, Belize*

Echocardiography Illustrated

Echo Stethoscope Academy Project

Longwood Medical and Academic Area

400 Brookline Avenue, Suite 23F

Boston, Massachusetts, USA, 02215

Contact: info@echoscope.org

Registered offices: Echo Stethoscope Academy Limited

Pitts and Associates

90 North Front Street

Belize City, P.O. Box 904

Belize, Central America

Books and products by Echo Stethoscope Academy are available on Amazon.com

Author: author@echoscope.org

Copyright © 2020 by Echo Stethoscope Academy Ltd.

All rights reserved. No part of the material protected by this copyright may be reproduced or utilized in any form, electronic or mechanical, including photocopying, recording, or by any information storage and retrieval system, without written permission from the copyright owner.

The author and publisher have made every effort to provide accurate information. However, they are not responsible for errors, omissions, or for any outcomes related to the use of the contents of this book and take no responsibility for the use of the products and procedures described. Medical devices are discussed that may have limited availability controlled by the Food and Drug Administration (FDA) for use only in a research study or clinical trial. Research, clinical practice, and government regulations often change the accepted standard in this field. When consideration is given to use of any device or drug in the clinical setting, the health care provider or reader is responsible for determining FDA status of the device or drug, reading the package insert, and reviewing prescribing information

Production Credits:

Publisher: Echo Stethoscope Academy, Inc.

Editor, Author, Illustrator, and Cover Design: Bernard E. Bulwer, M.D., FASE

Bulwer, Bernard E.

Echocardiography Illustrated Series:

Echocardiography Illustrated. Vol. 4; Coronary Artery Territories/ Bernard E. Bulwer. p. ; cm.

Includes bibliographical references and index.

ISBN-: 9798674132561

1. Echocardiography—Handbooks, manuals, etc. I. Bulwer, Bernard E. II. Title.

Printed in the United States of America

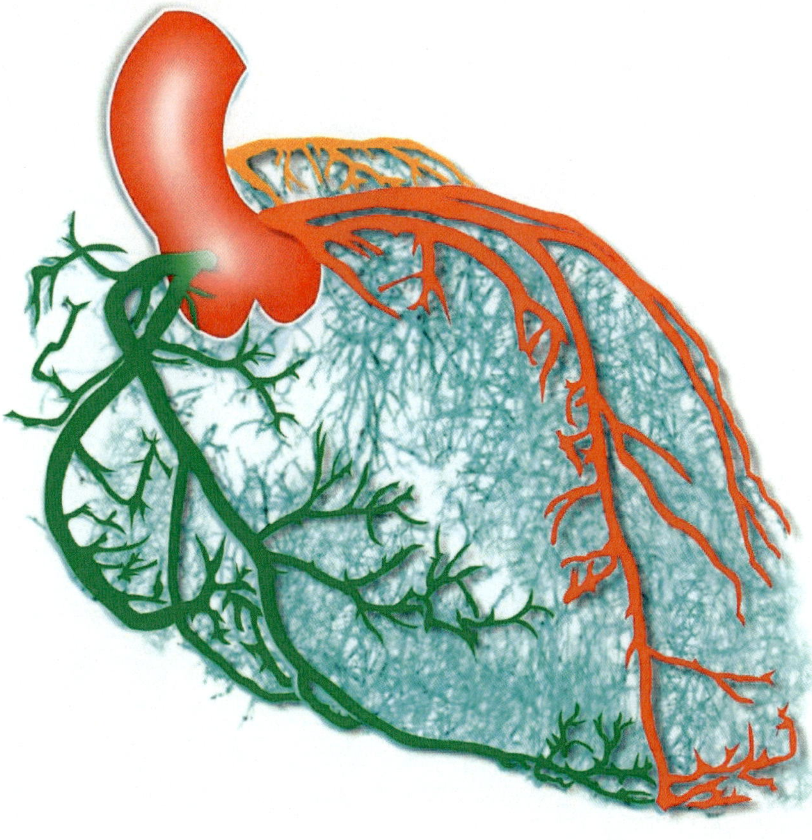

Coronary Artery Territories, Imaging Planes, and Left Ventricular Segments

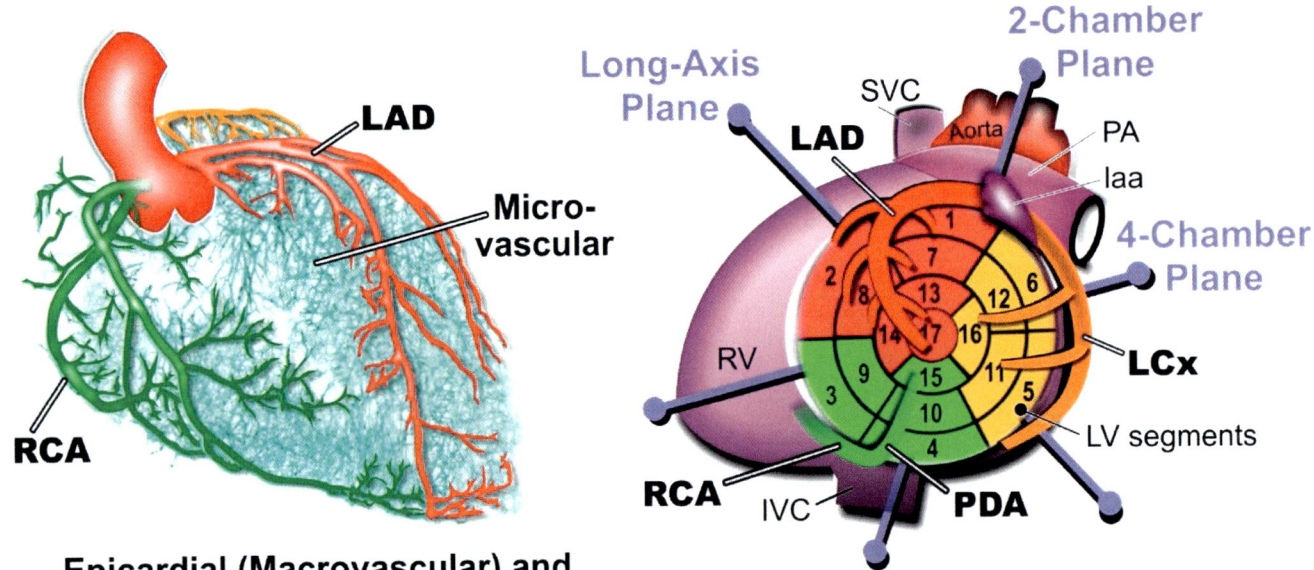

Epicardial (Macrovascular) and Microvascular Coronary Artery Territories

Polar "Bull's Eye" Plot
Left Anterior Oblique (LAO) View

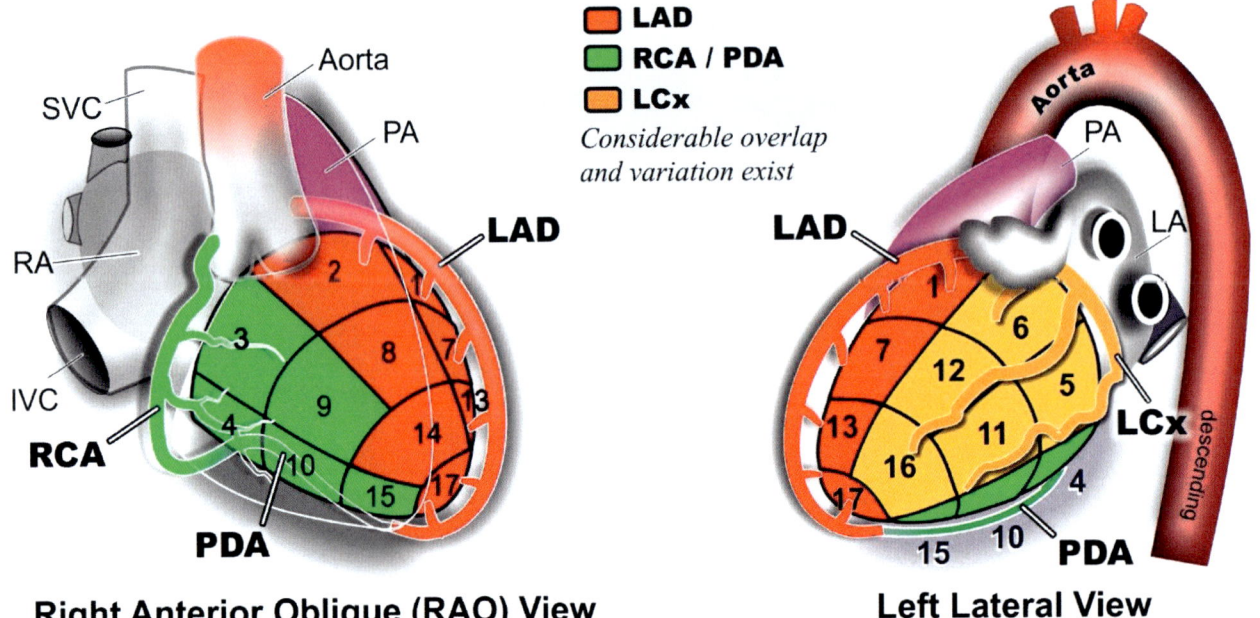

- LAD
- RCA / PDA
- LCx

Considerable overlap and variation exist

Right Anterior Oblique (RAO) View

Left Lateral View

Basal	Mid-LV	Apical	Apex
1. basal anterior	7. mid anterior	13. apical anterior	17. apex
2. basal anteroseptal	8. mid anteroseptal	14. apical septal	
3. basal inferoseptal	9. mid inferoseptal	15. apical inferior	
4. basal inferior	10. mid inferior	16. apical lateral	
5. basal inferolateral	11. mid inferolateral		
6. basal anterolateral	12. mid anterolatral		

BE Bulwer, MD, FASE

Left Ventricular (LV) Segments

LAD, left anterior descending coronary artery; **RCA/PDA**, right coronary and posteior descending artery; **LCA**, left circumflex artery

Coronary Artery Territories, Echocardiographic Imaging Planes, and Left Ventricular Segmentation

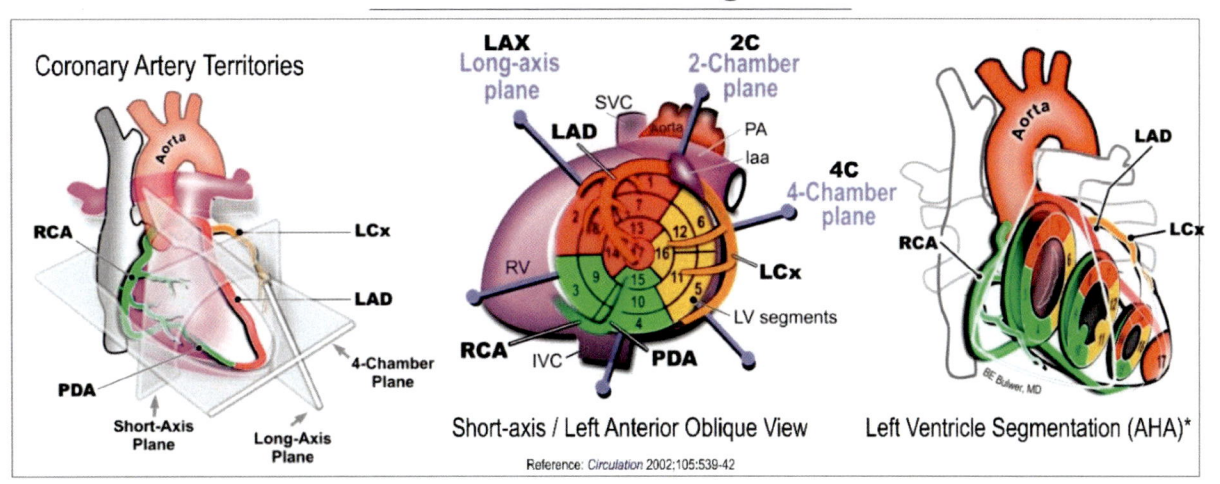

Coronary Artery Territories

Short-axis / Left Anterior Oblique View

Reference: *Circulation* 2002;105:539-42

Left Ventricle Segmentation (AHA)*

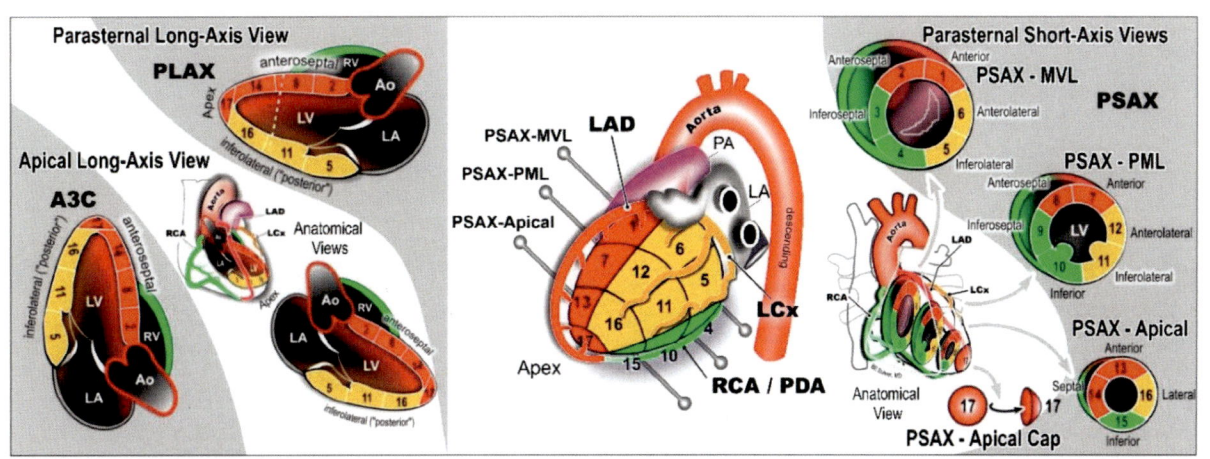

Long-Axis (LAX) Views

Parasternal Long-Axis View — PLAX
Apical Long-Axis View — A3C

Left Lateral View

Short-Axis (SAX) Views

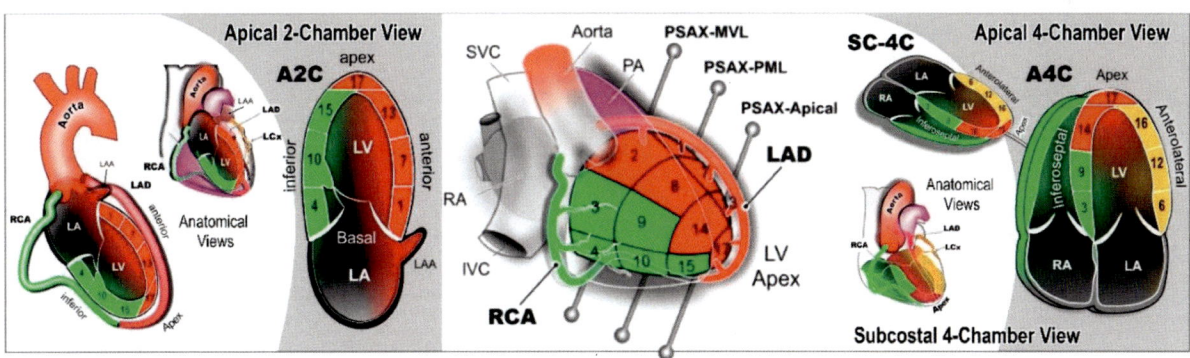

Parasternal Short-Axis Views
- PSAX - MVL
- PSAX - PML
- PSAX - Apical
- PSAX - Apical Cap

Apical Two-Chamber (A2C) View

Right Anterior Oblique (RAO) View

Four-Chamber (4C) Views

Apical 4-Chamber View — A4C
Subcostal 4-Chamber View — SC-4C

Left Ventricular (LV) Segments

BE Bulwer, MD, FASE

Coronary Arteries
- **LAD**: left anterior descending
- **LCx**: left circumflex branch
- **RCA / PDA**: right coronary / posterior descending artery

Considerable overlap and variation exist

Basal LV
1. basal anterior
2. basal anteroseptal
3. basal inferoseptal
4. basal inferior
5. basal inferolateral
6. basal anterolateral

Mid-LV
7. mid anterior
8. mid anteroseptal
9. mid inferoseptal
10. mid inferior
11. mid inferolateral
12. mid anterolateral

Apical LV
13. apical anterior
14. apical septal
15. apical inferior
16. apical lateral

LV Apex
17. apex

Standardized Myocardial Segmentation and Nomenclature. *Circulation* 2002;105:539-42

PLAX, Parasternal Long-Axis; **PSAX-MVL**, Parasternal Short-Axis (Mitral Valve Level); **PSAX-PML**, PSAX (Papillary Muscle or Mid-LV Level); **PSAX-Apical**, PSAX (Apical level); **A4C**, Apical 4-Chamber View; **A2C**, Apical 2-Chamber View; **A3C / ALAX**, Apical 3-Chamber or Apical Long-Axis View

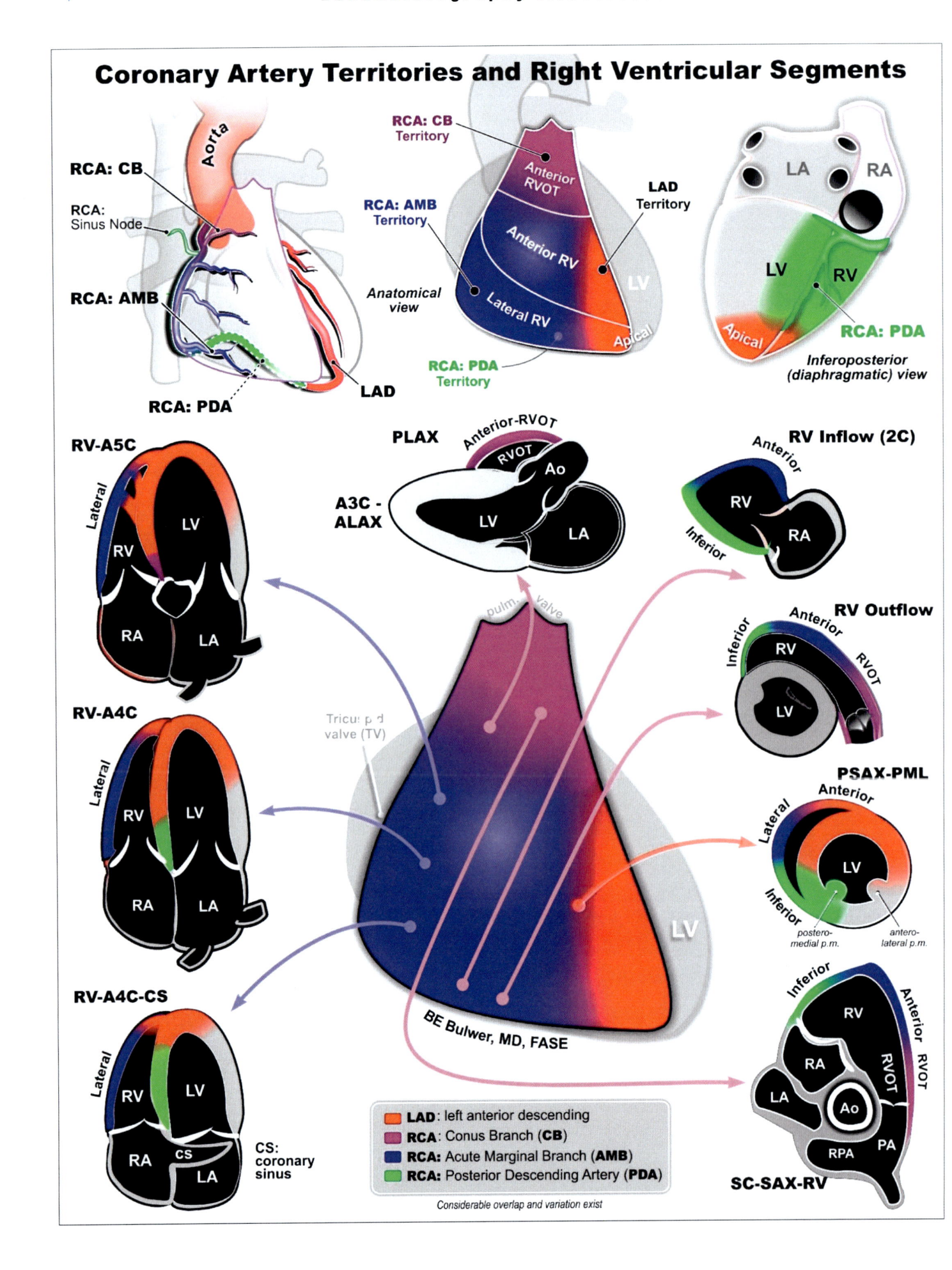

Coronary Artery Territories and Right Ventricular Segments

Echocardiography Illustrated

LAD: left anterior descending
RCA: Conus Branch (**CB**)
RCA: Acute Marginal Branch (**AMB**)
RCA: Posterior Descending Artery (**PDA**)

Considerable overlap and variation exist

BE Bulwer, MD, FASE

Table Of Contents

Table Of Contents 1
Coronary Artery Territories And Echo Imaging Planes 5
Coronary Artery Anatomy 6
Two-Dimensional Adult Echocardiography Protocol 7
Coronary Artery Territories And Echo Imaging Planes 8
Coronary Artery Territories And Lv Segmentation I 9
Coronary Artery Territories And Lv Segmentation Ii 10
Coronary Artery Territories And Lv Segmentation Iii 11
Coronary Artery Territories And Lv Segmentation Iv 12
Coronary Artery Anatomy: Angiographic Views 13
Plax View, Lv Walls, And Coronary Artery Supply 14
Plax View, Lv Segments, And Coronary Artery Supply 15
The Aorta, Aortic Root, And Coronary Arteries I 16
The Aorta, Aortic Root, And Coronary Arteries Ii 17
Psax-Pulmonary Artery Bifurcation And Coronary Arteries 18
Psax Views, Aortic Root, And Coronary Arteries 19
Psax-Aortic Valve Level And Coronary Arteries 20
Psax Scan Planes And Corresponding Anatomy 21
Tee Of The Aortic Valve And Coronary Arteries 22
Psax View-Mitral Valve Level And Basal Lv Segments 23
Psax Views-Mid Lv And Apical Lv Segments 24
Psax Views, Lv Segments, And Coronary Artery Supply 25
A4c View, Lv Walls, And Coronary Artery Supply 26
A4c View, Lv Segments, And Coronary Artery Supply 27
A2c View, Lv Walls, And Coronary Artery Supply 28
A2c View, Lv Segments, And Coronary Artery Supply 29
A3c View, Lv Walls, And Coronary Artery Supply 30
A3c View, Lv Segments, And Coronary Artery Supply 31
Wall Motion Abnormalities: Ischemic Vs. Nonischemic 32

Ischemic Cascade: Utility Of Echocardiography 33

Coronary Microvasculature And Clinical Correlates I 34

Coronary Microvasculature And Clinical Correlates Ii 35

Coronary Ischemia And Wall Motion Assessment 36

Wall Motion Assessment In Stress Echocardiography I 37

Wall Motion Assessment In Stress Echocardiography Ii 38

Stress Echocardiography: Utility And Indications 39

Global Echo Measures Of Myocardial Ischemia I 40

Global Echo Measures Of Myocardial Ischemia Ii 41

Deformation Parameters In Myocardial Ischemia I 42

Deformation Parameters In Myocardial Ischemia Ii... 43

Echo Modality Options In Myocardial Assessment I 44

Echo Modality Options In Myocardial Assessment Ii 45

Global Longitudinal Lv Strain And Strain Rate I... 46

Global Longitudinal Lv Strain And Strain Rate Ii... 47

Tdi-Derived Global Longitudinal Strain Rate I 48

Tdi-Derived Global Longitudinal Strain Rate Ii 49

Tdi-Derived Measures Of Systolic Function I.. 50

Myocardial Longitudinal Strain And Strain Rate I 51

Myocardial Longitudinal Strain And Strain Rate Ii 52

Strain And Strain Rate: Longitudinal, Radial, Circumferential 53

Myocardial Velocities And Display Options I 54

Ste-Based Myocardial Velocities And Display Options Ii... 55

Longitudinal, Radial, And Circumferential Strain I 56

Longitudinal, Radial, And Circumferential Strain Ii 57

Circumferential Strain And Strain Rate I 58

Global Longitudinal Strain: "Bull's Eye" Plot... 59

Lv Strain Imaging: Clinical Applications 60

Coronary Artery Territories And Ischemic Patterns I 61

Coronary Artery Territories And Ischemic Patterns Ii 62

- Coronary Artery Territories And Ischemic Patterns Iii 63
- Global And Regional Longitudinal Strain 64
- Global Strain, Dyssynchrony, And Resynchronization 65
- Regional Wall Motion Assessment 66
- Post-Infarction Lv Remodeling And Volume Changes 67
- Coronary Artery Anatomy And The Right Ventricle 69
- 3d Echocardiographic Anatomy 70
- 2d Echo Assessment Of The Right Ventricle I 71
- 2d Echo Assessment Of The Right Ventricle Ii 72
- 2d Echo Assessment Of The Right Ventricle Iii 73
- 2d Echo Assessment Of The Right Ventricle Iv 74
- Coronary Arteries Supply To The Right Ventricle I 75
- Coronary Arteries Supply To The Right Ventricle Ii 76
- Coronary Arteries Supply To The Right Ventricle Iii 77
- Coronary Arteries Supply To The Right Ventricle Iv 78
- Coronary Arteries Supply To The Right Ventricle V 79
- Coronary Arteries Supply To The Right Ventricle Vi 80
- Coronary Arteries Supply To The Right Ventricle Vii 81
- Coronary Artery Assessment By Myocardial Contrast Echocardiography 82
- Ultrasound Contrast Agents: Basic Properties 83
- Ultrasound Contrast Agents: Physical Principles 84
- Clinical Utility Of Contrast Agents In Echocardiography I 85
- Contrast Echocardiography: Optimizing Image Acquisition 86
- Myocardial Blood Flow Using Contrast Ultrasound 87
- References 88
- Glossary: Abbreviations And Symbols 90

Coronary Artery Territories and Echo Imaging Planes

Coronary artery disease (CAD) is a leading cause of morbidity and mortality worldwide. Knowledge of the blood supply to the heart, especially to the ventricular myocardium, is a requisite for the echocardiographic assessment of patients with coronary artery disease (Figs. 1-80).

The coronary circulation includes both arterial supply and venous drainage, but our focus here is the arterial supply via the left and right coronary arteries that arise from their respective coronary sinuses within the aortic root. These large epicardial coronary arteries descend in a corona-like fashion along the atrioventricular and interventricular grooves, just below the epicardium, progressively branching to supply the myocardium and epicardium. Varying degrees of collateral circulation exists within the coronary circulation, especially at the microvascular level (Figs. 1-9; 29-32).

Coronary artery disease is a major cause of ventricular or regional wall motion abnormalities (RWMA), ventricular dysfunction, and ventricular remodeling following ischemic insults to the myocardium (Figs. 28-80).

The ventricular wall segments, which are artificial subdivisions of the ventricular walls by convention, represent myocardial territories variously supplied by the coronary arteries (Figs. 3-27). This is the basis for the parametric displays and semiquantitative assessment of RWMA in patients with coronary artery disease, including stress echocardiography (Figs. 28-34, 40, 54-61; Table 1).

Ventricular walls that demonstrate RWMA, i.e., abnormal movement and thickening, e.g. hypokinesis, akinesis, or dyskinesis, and ventricular walls that appear aneurysmal, or thinned (or scarred), do so most commonly because of insults to their corresponding coronary artery supply (Figs. 28-34, 59-62; Table 1). Regional wall motion abnormalities in the acute setting is strong evidence to support the diagnosis of acute coronary syndromes.

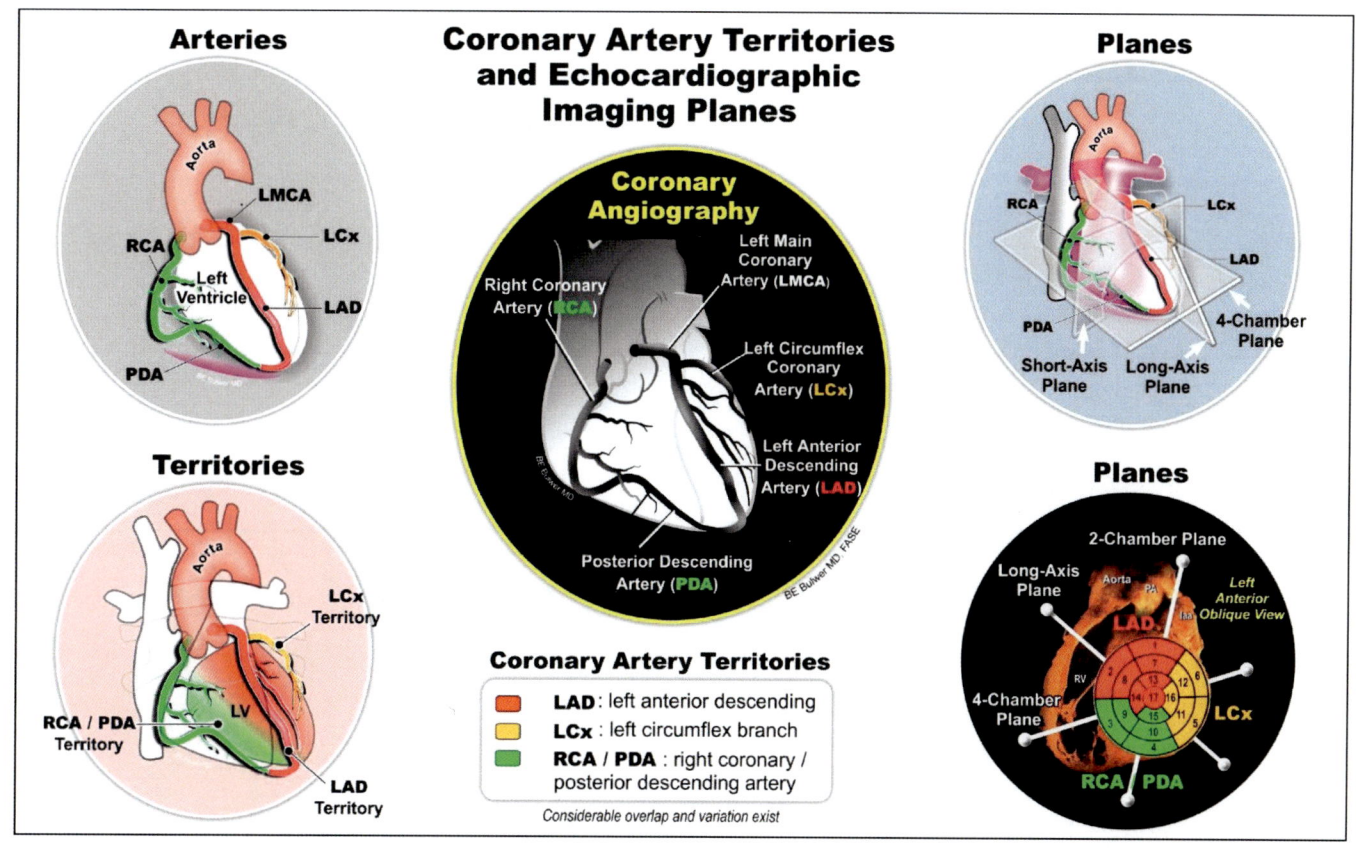

Fig. 1. The epicardial coronary arteries and their relationship to the echocardiographic imaging planes. LAA: left atrial appendage; **LAD:** left anterior descending coronary artery; **LCx:** left circumflex coronary artery; LMA: left main coronary artery; **PDA:** posterior descending (branch of the right coronary) artery; **RCA:** right coronary artery.

Coronary Artery Anatomy

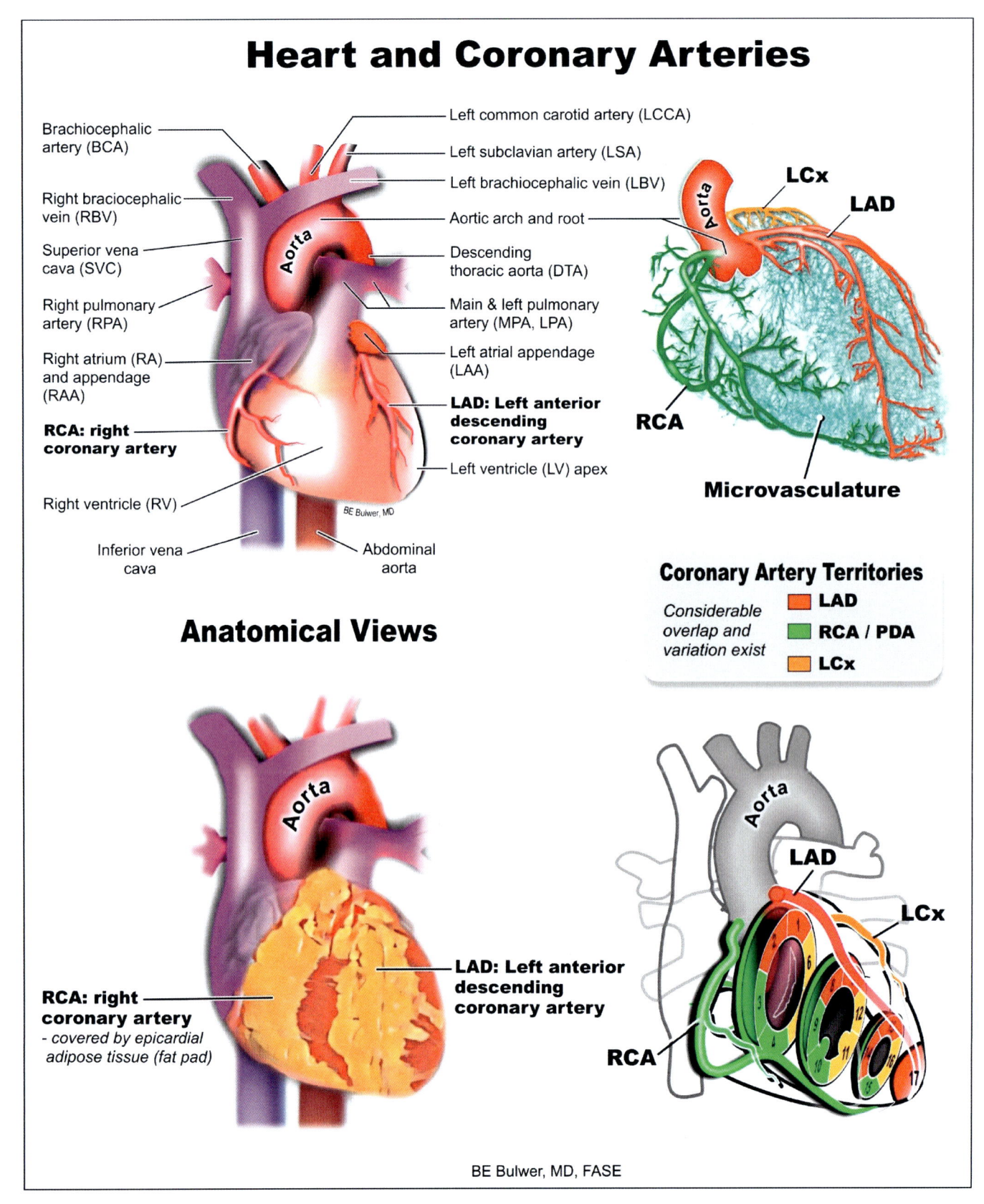

Fig. 2. **Anatomical perspectives of the heart, showing the major coronary arteries.** Note the origins and course of the right and left coronary arteries. The major coronary vessels course along the atrioventricular and interventricular grooves, just below the epicardium, and typically covered in epicardial adipose tissue. Compare with Figs. 1-27.

Two-Dimensional Adult Echocardiography Protocol

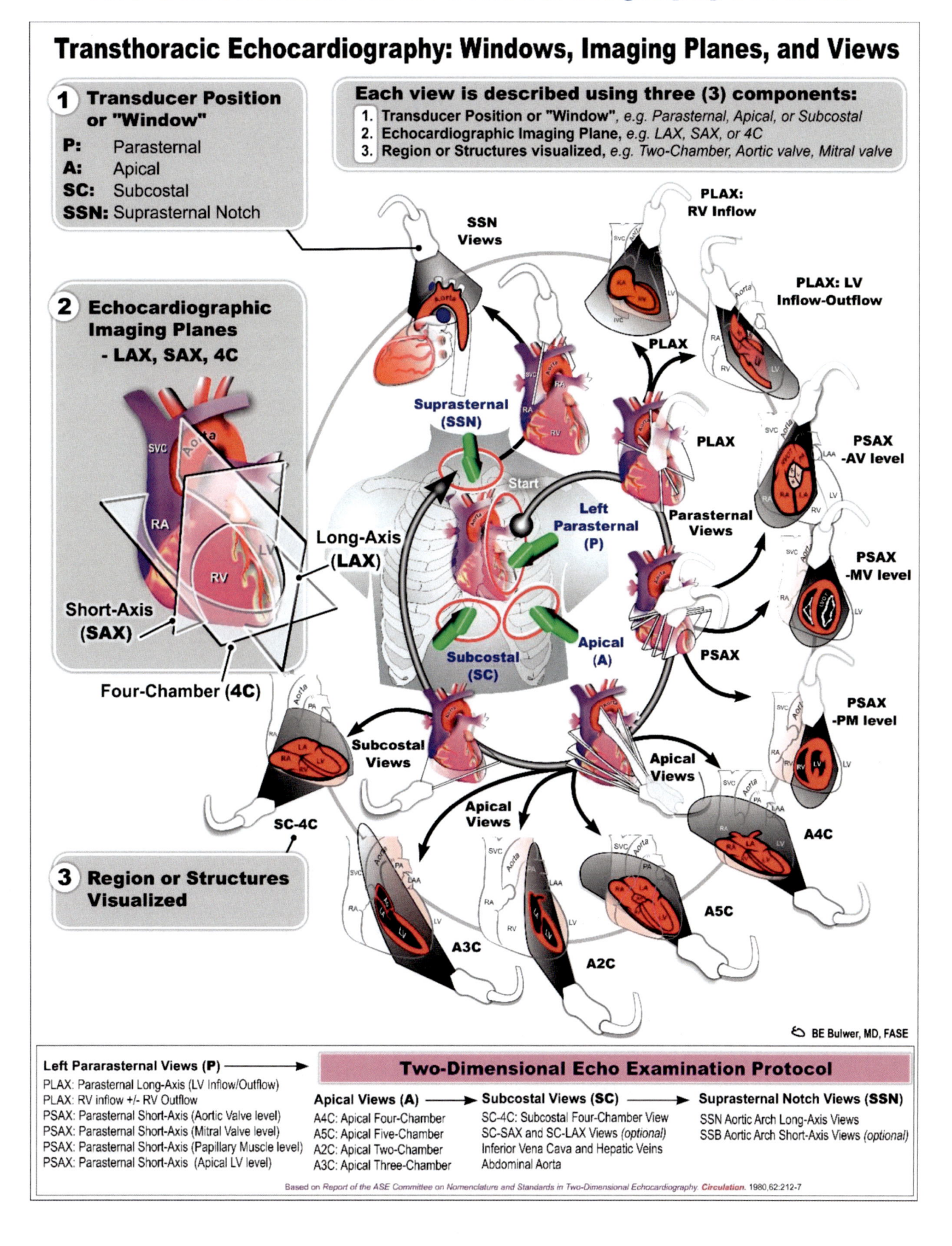

Transthoracic Echocardiography: Windows, Imaging Planes, and Views

1. Transducer Position or "Window"
- **P:** Parasternal
- **A:** Apical
- **SC:** Subcostal
- **SSN:** Suprasternal Notch

Each view is described using three (3) components:
1. Transducer Position or "Window", e.g. Parasternal, Apical, or Subcostal
2. Echocardiographic Imaging Plane, e.g. LAX, SAX, or 4C
3. Region or Structures visualized, e.g. Two-Chamber, Aortic valve, Mitral valve

2. Echocardiographic Imaging Planes - LAX, SAX, 4C
- Long-Axis (LAX)
- Short-Axis (SAX)
- Four-Chamber (4C)

3. Region or Structures Visualized

Views shown: SSN Views, PLAX: RV Inflow, PLAX: LV Inflow-Outflow, PLAX, PSAX -AV level, PSAX -MV level, PSAX -PM level, A4C, A5C, A2C, A3C, SC-4C, Subcostal Views, Apical Views, Parasternal Views, Suprasternal (SSN), Left Parasternal (P), Subcostal (SC), Apical (A), Start

© BE Bulwer, MD, FASE

Two-Dimensional Echo Examination Protocol

Left Parasternal Views (P)
- PLAX: Parasternal Long-Axis (LV Inflow/Outflow)
- PLAX: RV inflow +/- RV Outflow
- PSAX: Parasternal Short-Axis (Aortic Valve level)
- PSAX: Parasternal Short-Axis (Mitral Valve level)
- PSAX: Parasternal Short-Axis (Papillary Muscle level)
- PSAX: Parasternal Short-Axis (Apical LV level)

Apical Views (A)
- A4C: Apical Four-Chamber
- A5C: Apical Five-Chamber
- A2C: Apical Two-Chamber
- A3C: Apical Three-Chamber

Subcostal Views (SC)
- SC-4C: Subcostal Four-Chamber View
- SC-SAX and SC-LAX Views (optional)
- Inferior Vena Cava and Hepatic Veins
- Abdominal Aorta

Suprasternal Notch Views (SSN)
- SSN Aortic Arch Long-Axis Views
- SSB Aortic Arch Short-Axis Views (optional)

Based on Report of the ASE Committee on Nomenclature and Standards in Two-Dimensional Echocardiography. *Circulation*. 1980;62:212-7

Coronary Artery Territories and Echo Imaging Planes

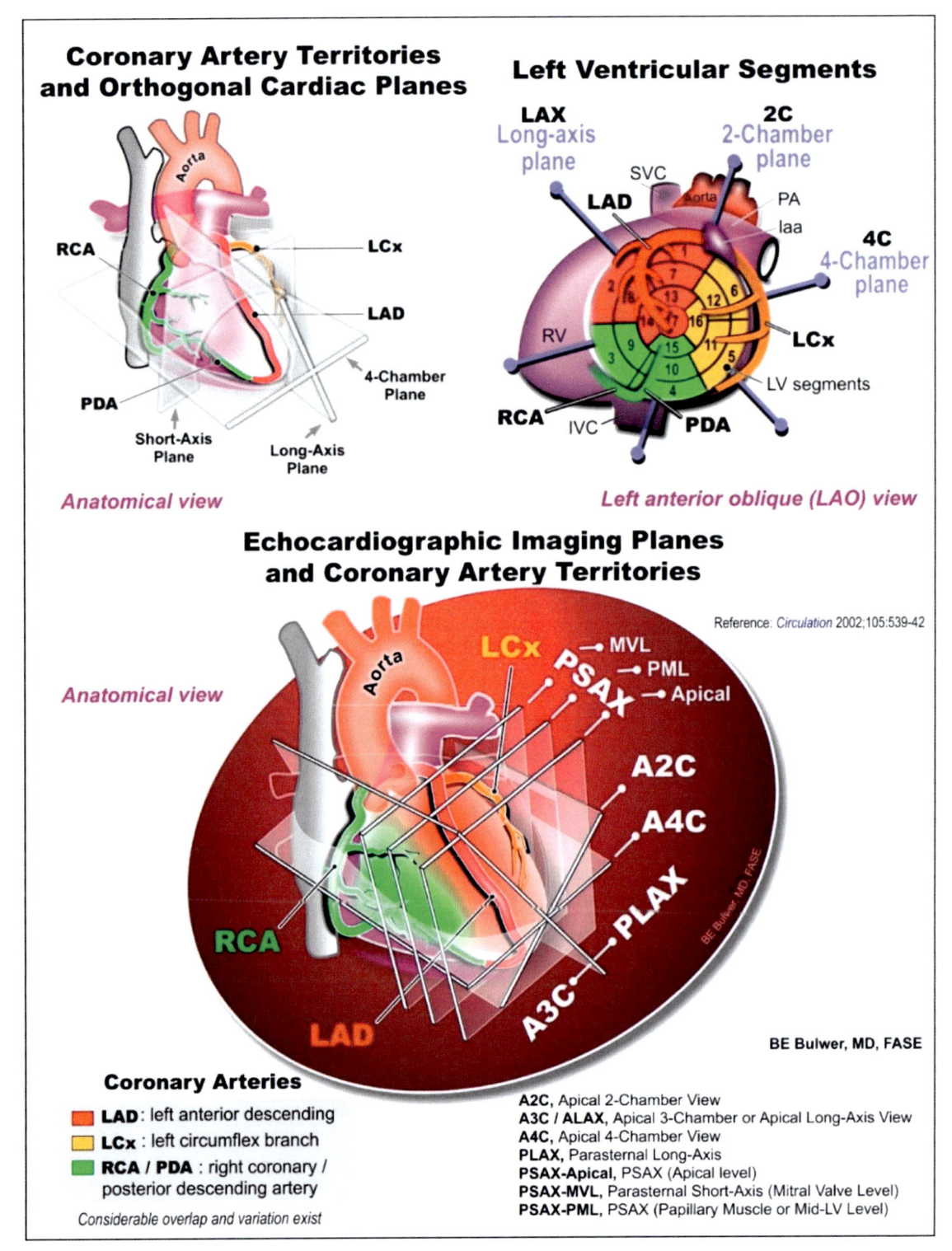

Fig. 4. Echocardiographic imaging planes with respect to the coronary arteries and myocardial territories. Compare with Figs. 5-27.

Fig. 3 *(Previous page).* In the comprehensive two-dimensional (2D) transthoracic echocardiography (TTE) protocol, as recommended by the American Society of Echocardiography (ASE), **each component echocardiographic view is described using three (3) parameters: (i) transducer position, (ii) echocardiographic imaging plane, and (iii) region or structures visualized.** The adult TTE examination protocol begins at the left parasternal window (P), followed by examination at the subsequent windows *(green arrows).*

Coronary Artery Territories and LV Segmentation I

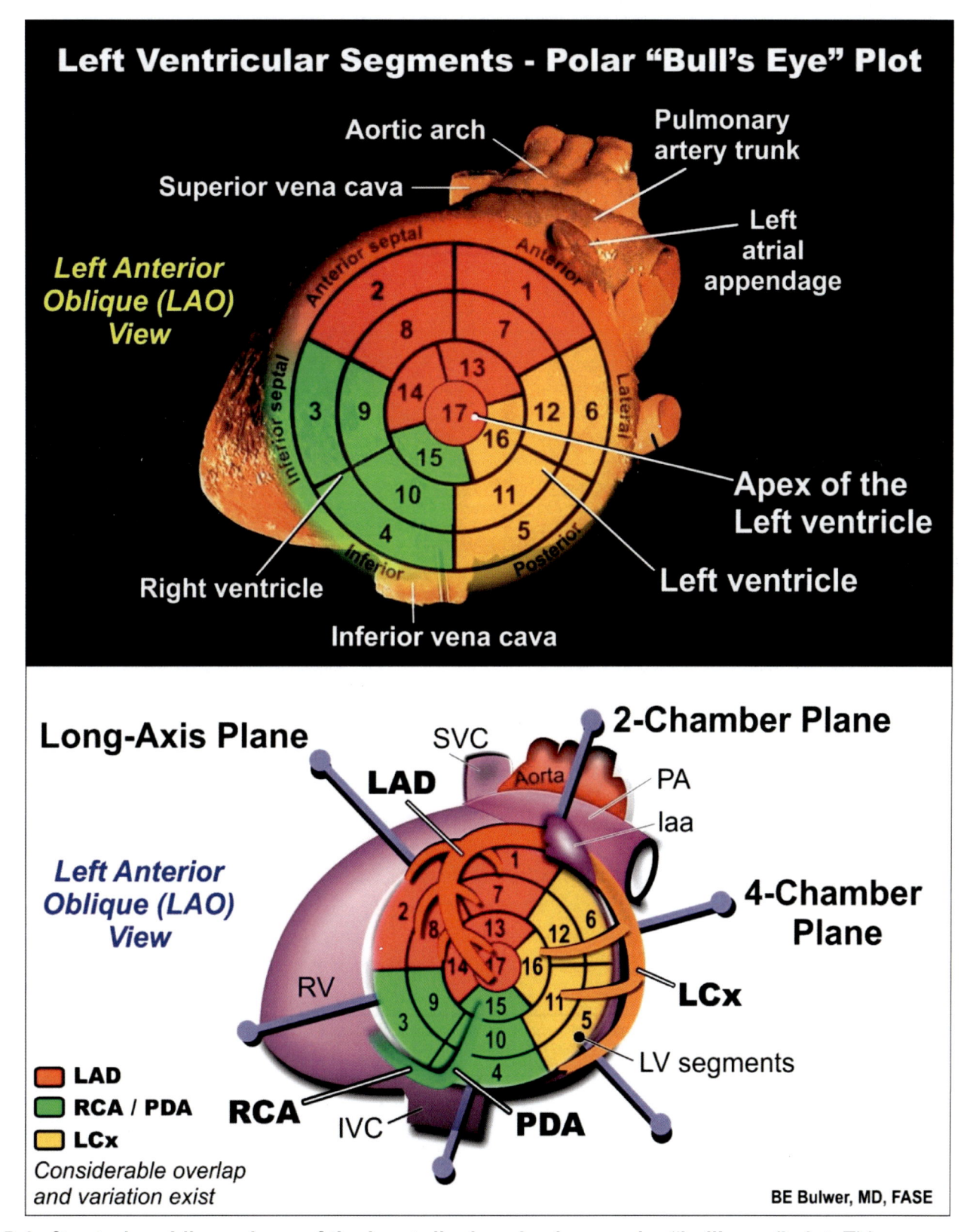

Fig 5. Left anterior oblique views of the heart displayed using a polar "bull's eye" plot. This nomenclature numbers **the left ventricular (LV) myocardial segments from 1 to 17**, with the six **basal LV segments numbered 1-6**, the six **mid LV segments 7-12**, the four **apical segments 13-16**, and the **apical cap numbered 17**. Correlate with Figs. 4-27.

Coronary Artery Territories and LV Segmentation II

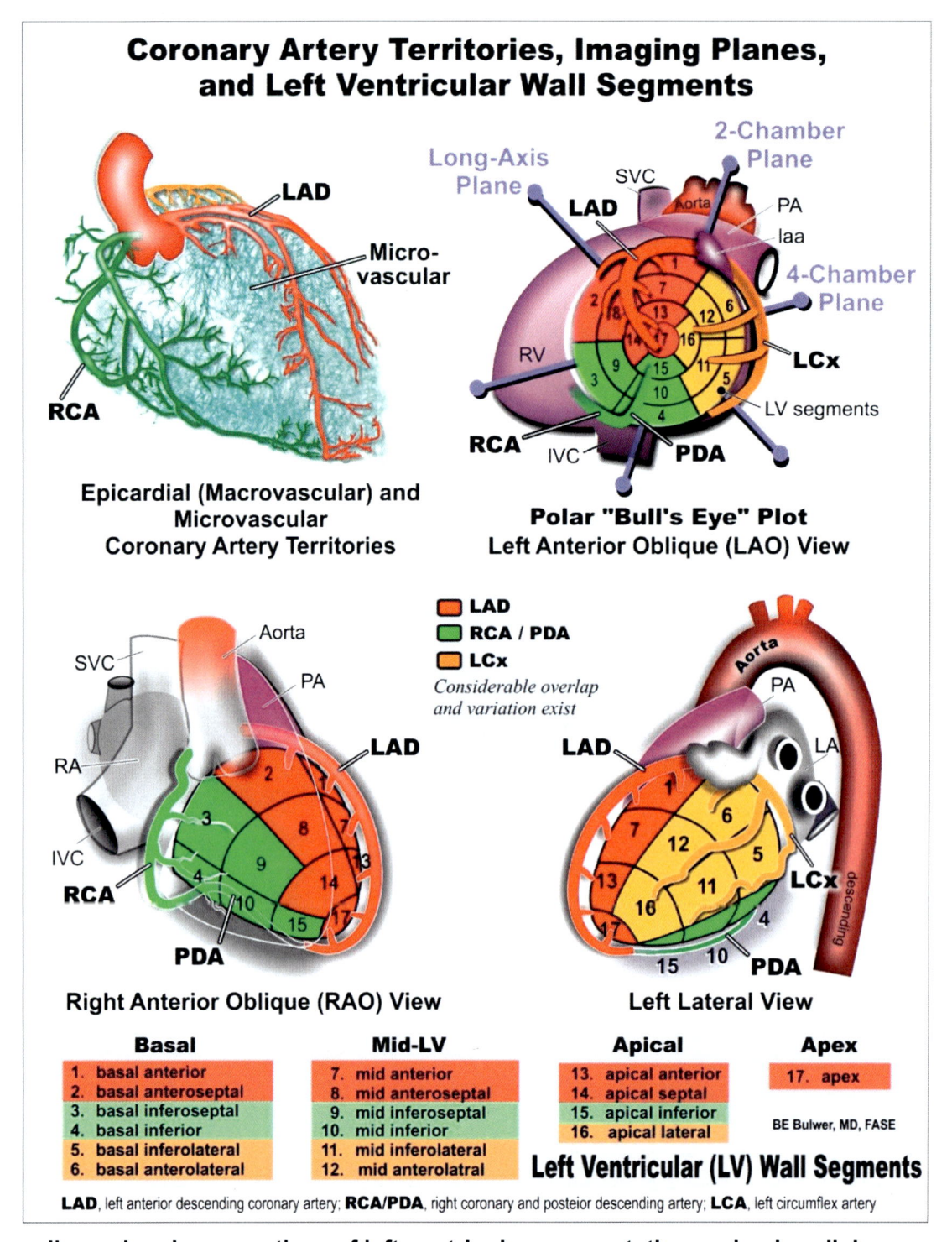

Fig. 6. Three-dimensional perspectives of left ventricular segmentation and epicardial coronary artery supply. Note the polar or "bull's eye" plot *(top)* based on standards set by expert groups, including the American Society of Echocardiography (ASE). Much variation and overlap exist in coronary artery supply. Complementary projections of the LV segments and their corresponding coronary artery territories *(bottom)*.

Fig. 7. *(See next page).* **Left ventricular (LV) segments, their corresponding coronary artery territories and echocardiographic views.** Correlation of regional wall motion abnormalities of the LV segments and their corresponding coronary blood supply is important in the echocardiographic assessment of ischemic heart disease, including stress echocardiographic interpretation. Compare with Figs. 4-76.

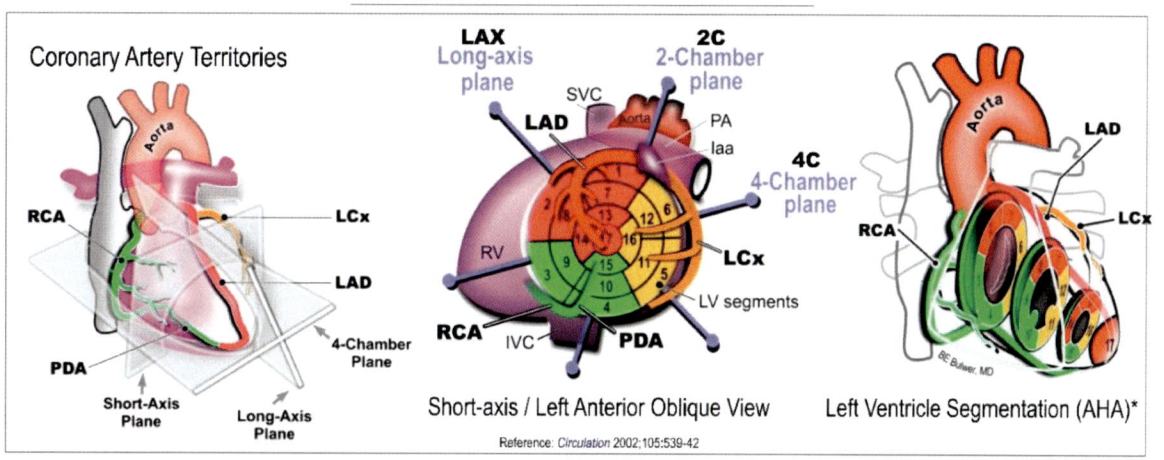

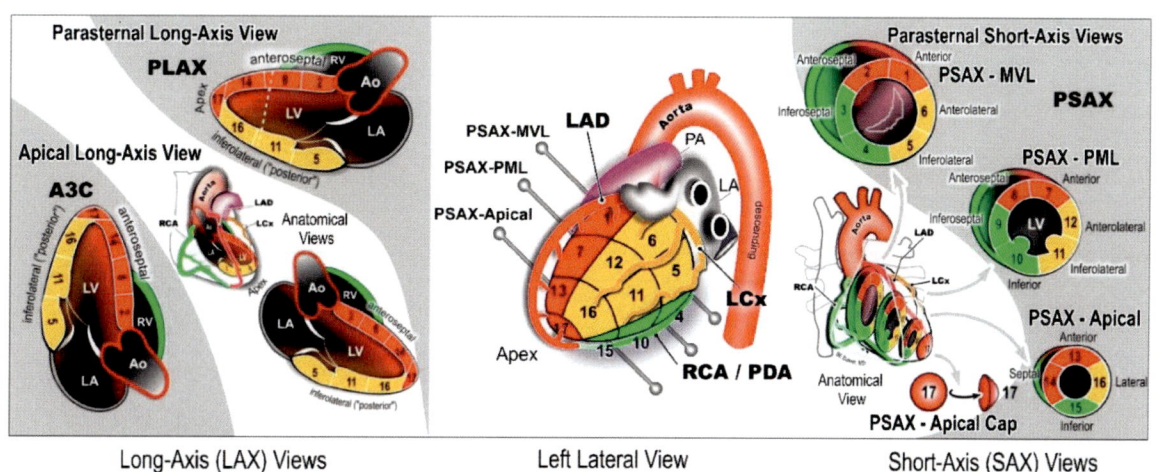

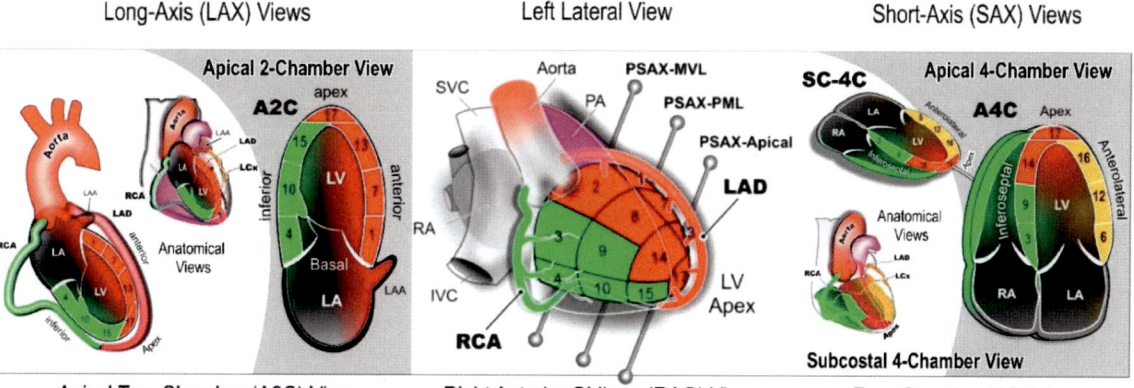

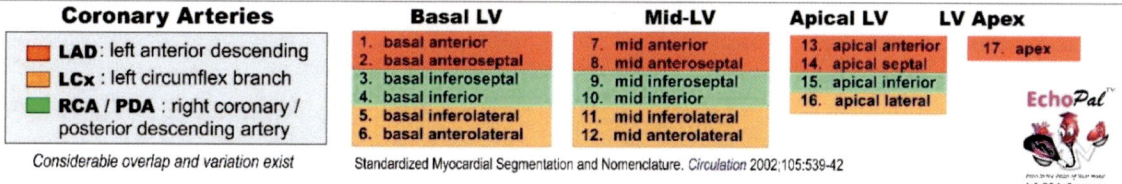

Coronary Artery Territories and LV Segmentation III

Coronary Artery Territories and LV Segmentation IV

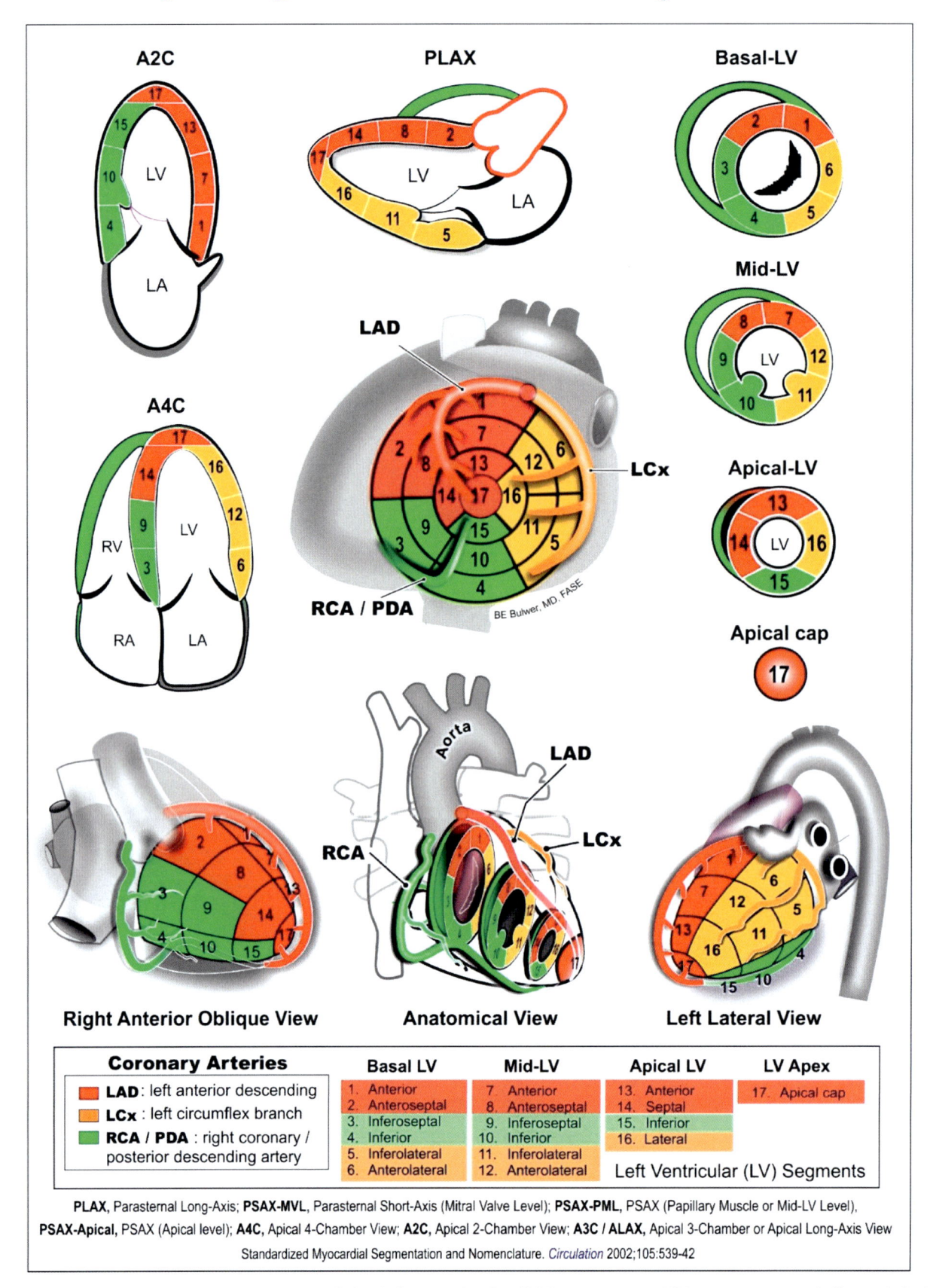

Fig. 8. Standard echocardiographic views of the left ventricular (LV) segments (17-segment model), and their corresponding coronary artery territories.

Coronary Artery Anatomy: Angiographic Views

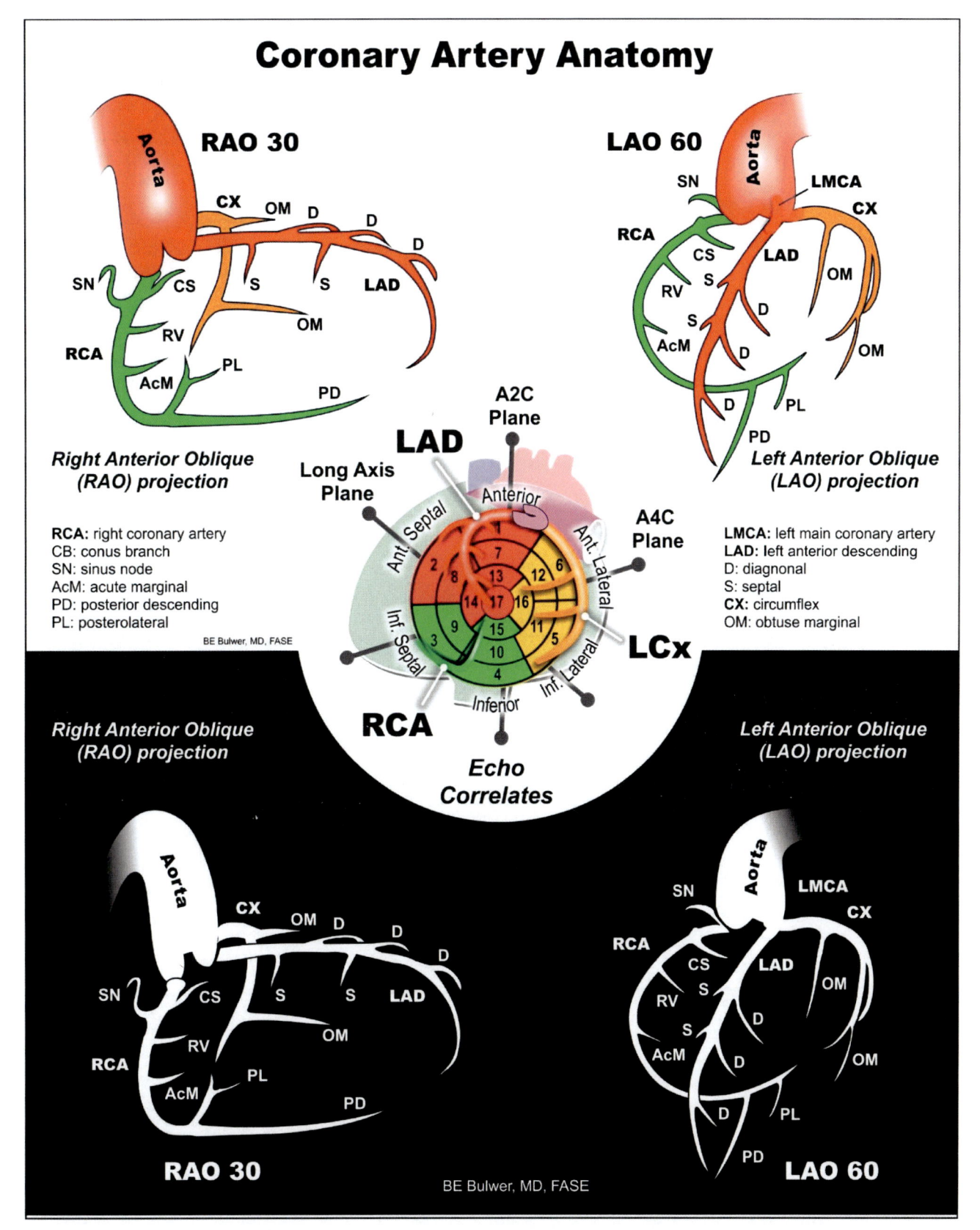

Fig. 9. Right anterior oblique (RAO) and the left anterior oblique (LAO) projections of the major coronary arteries and branches as displayed on coronary angiography. Note their relationship to the LV segmentation (17-segment model) used in echocardiography (insert). **Compare with** Figs. 1-8.

PLAX View, LV Walls, and Coronary Artery Supply

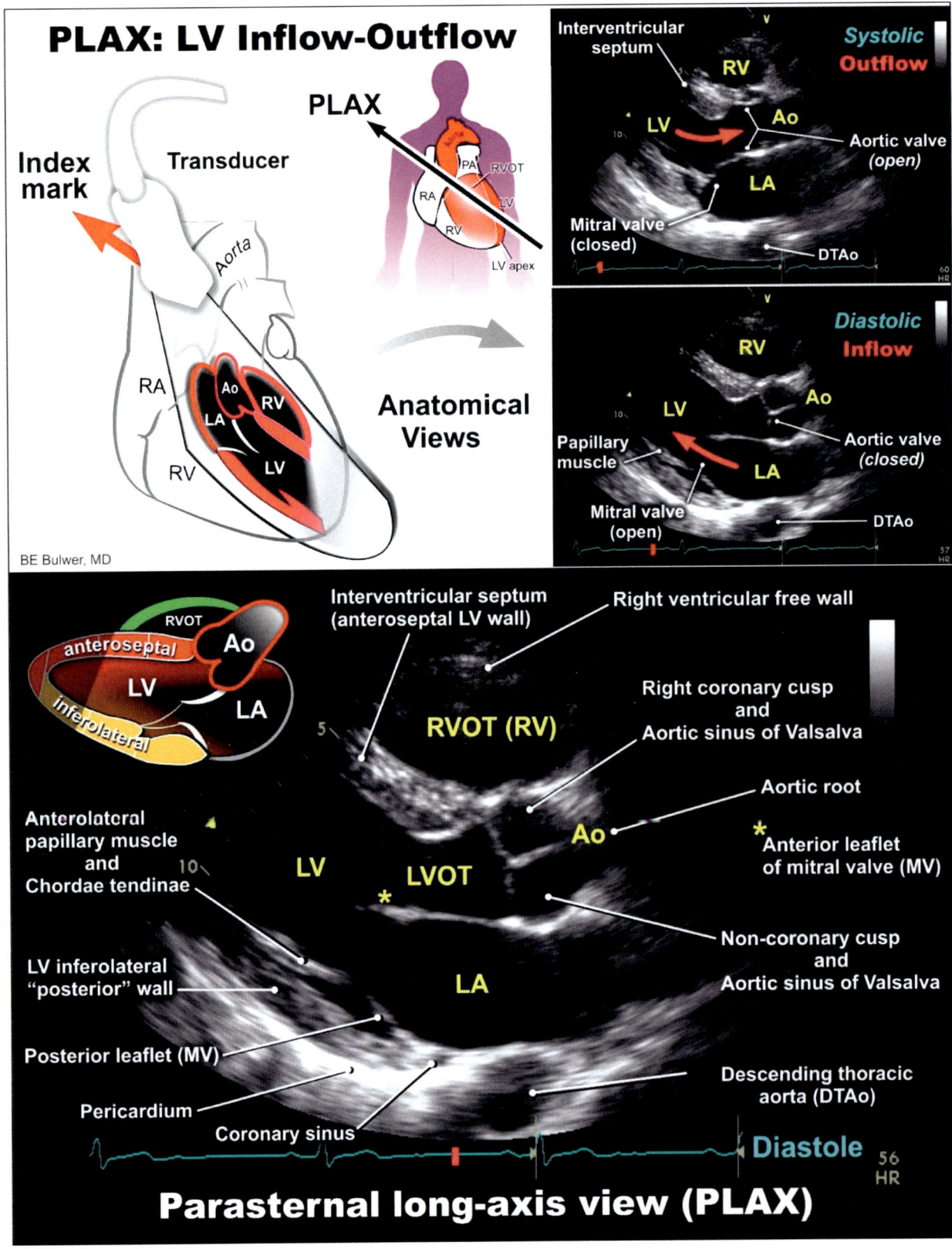

Fig 10. Parasternal long-axis (PLAX) view showing the anteroseptal wall (interventricular septum) and the inferolateral (posterior) wall of the left ventricle (LV). These walls, corresponding to the LV segments depicted in Fig. 11, are normally supplied by the left anterior descending (LAD) and the left circumflex (LCx) coronary arteries as shown. Compare with Figs. 1-8, 26, 32-34.

Coronary Artery Territories

PLAX View, LV Segments, and Coronary Artery Supply

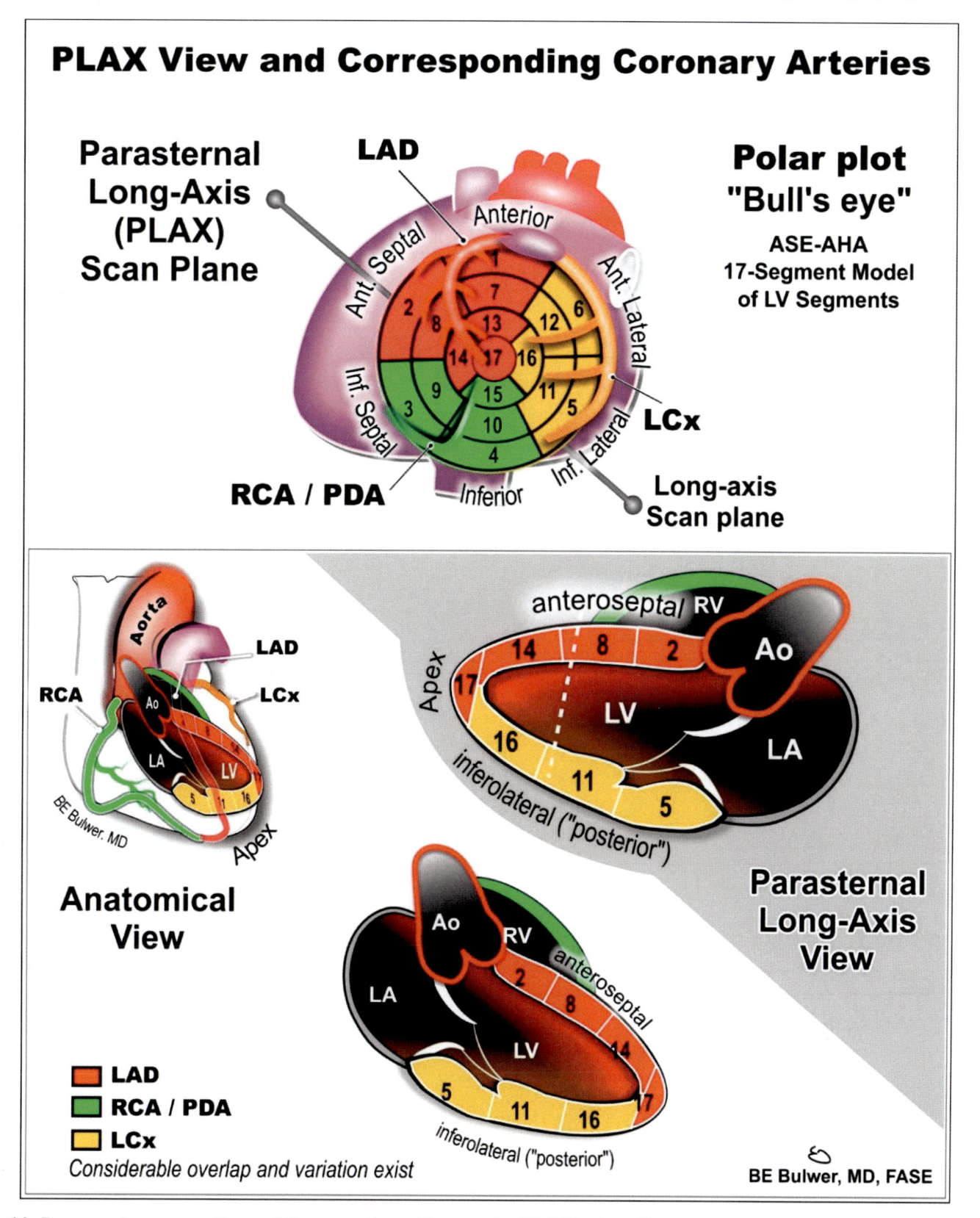

Fig 11. Panoramic perspectives of the parasternal long-axis (PLAX) view, the corresponding left ventricular (LV) segments, and their coronary artery supply. The same LV segments on the PLAX view are also seen on the apical long-axis view (ALAX), commonly called the apical three-chamber (A3C) view. However, unlike the ALAX view, the PLAX view does not include the LV apical segments. Compare with Figs. 1-8, 26, 27, 56-58).

The Aorta, Aortic Root, and Coronary Arteries I

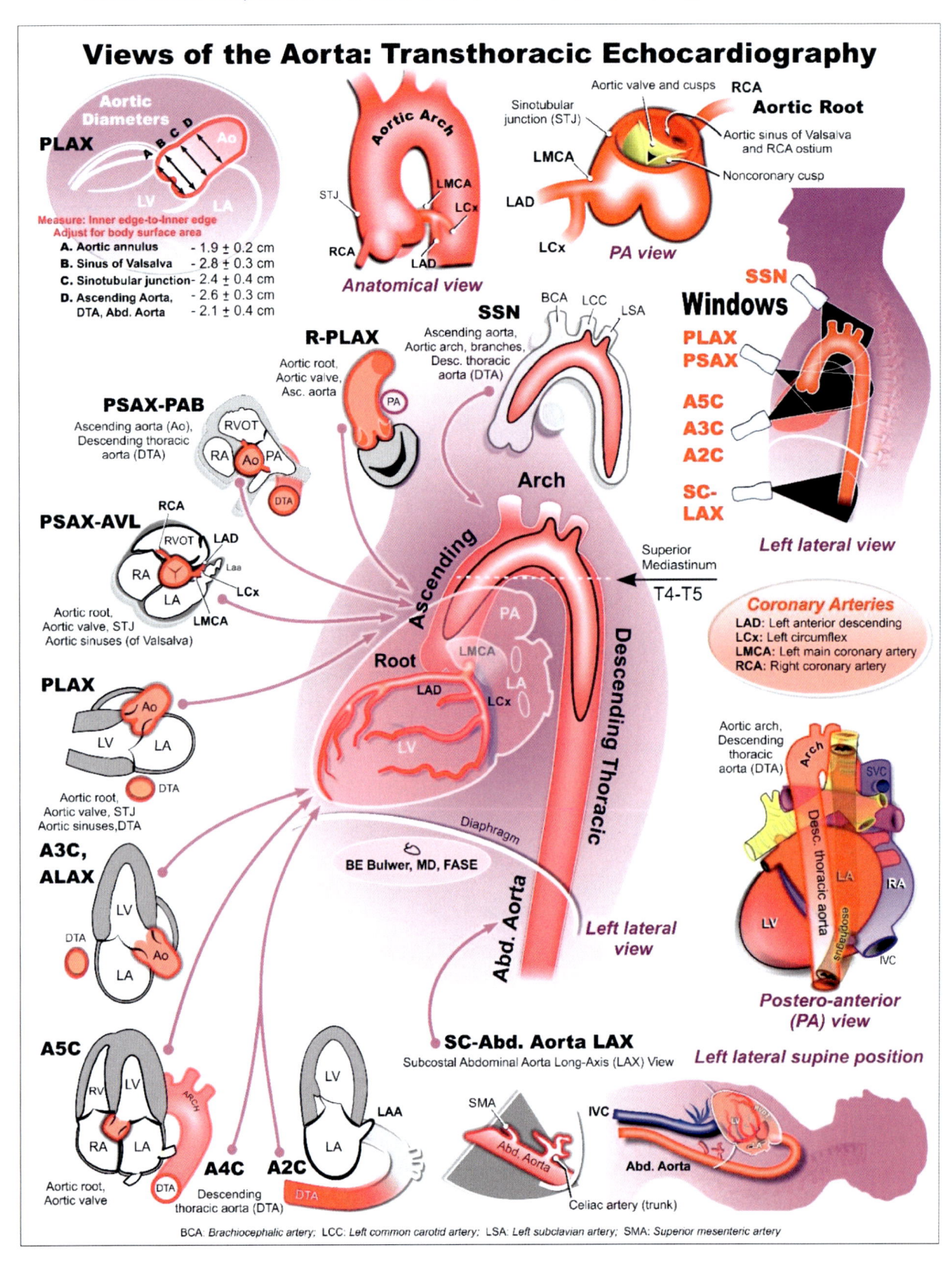

Fig 12. Echocardiographic views of the aorta, the aortic valve, and coronary arteries. Note the echocardiographic views used to examine the aortic root, from which the coronary arteries arise. The origins of the coronary arteries are often visible on the PSAX-AVL and PSAX-PAB views. Compare with Figs. 1-17.

The Aorta, Aortic Root, and Coronary Arteries II

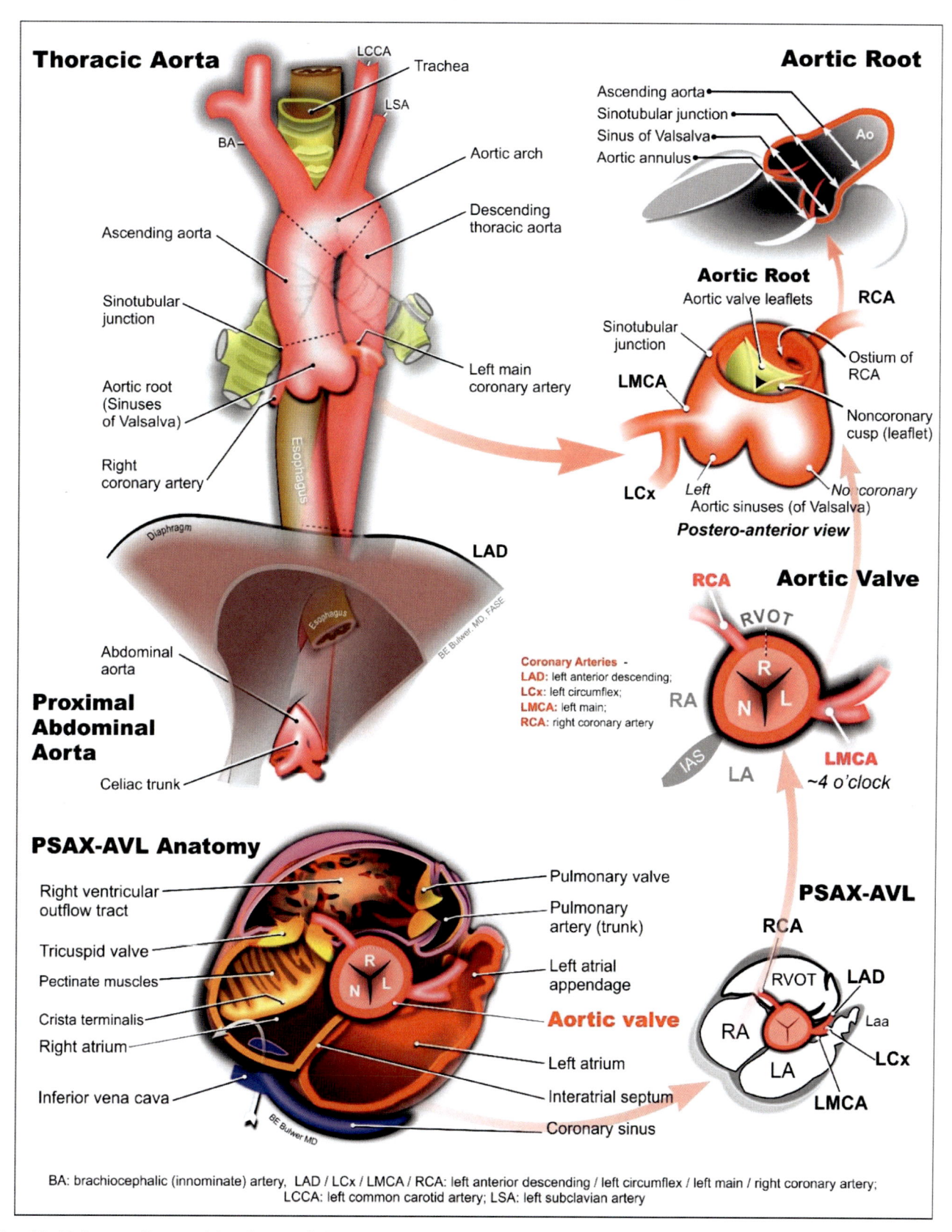

Fig. 13. Echocardiographic views of the thoracic aorta, the aortic valve, and coronary arteries arising from the aortic sinuses of Valsalva. The three aortic sinuses are anatomic dilatations of the aortic root, from which the **left main coronary (LMCA)** and **right coronary (RCA) arteries arise.** Note their anatomical orientation at ~4 o'clock and ~10 o'clock positions on the PSAX-AVL cross-sectional plane. Compare with Figs. 1-17.

PSAX-Pulmonary Artery Bifurcation and Coronary Arteries

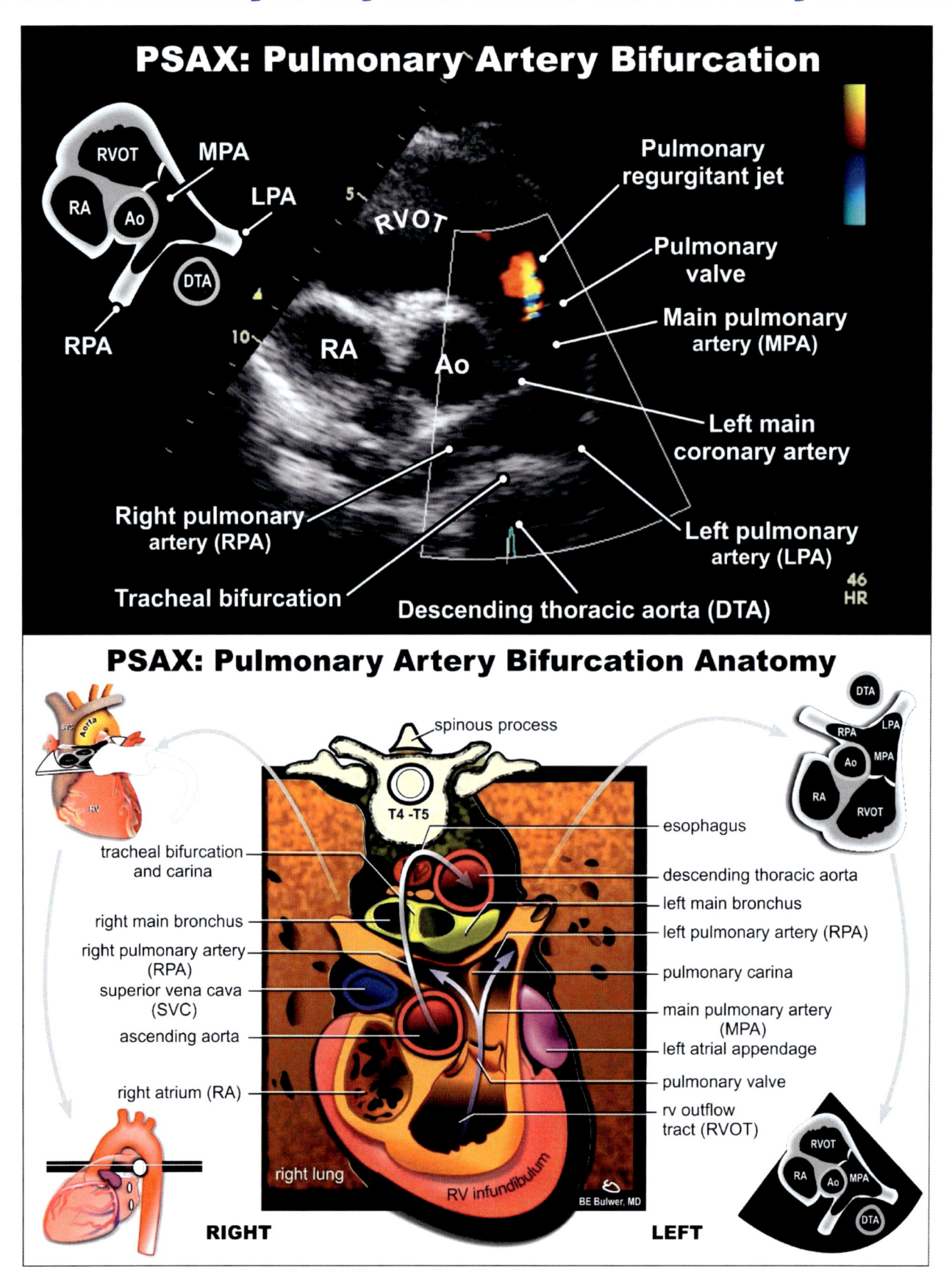

Fig. 14. Parasternal short-axis view and cross-sectional anatomy at the level of the pulmonary artery bifurcation (PSAX-PAB). Note the origin of the left main coronary artery (above). Compare with Figs. 1-17.

Coronary Artery Territories

PSAX Views, Aortic Root, and Coronary Arteries

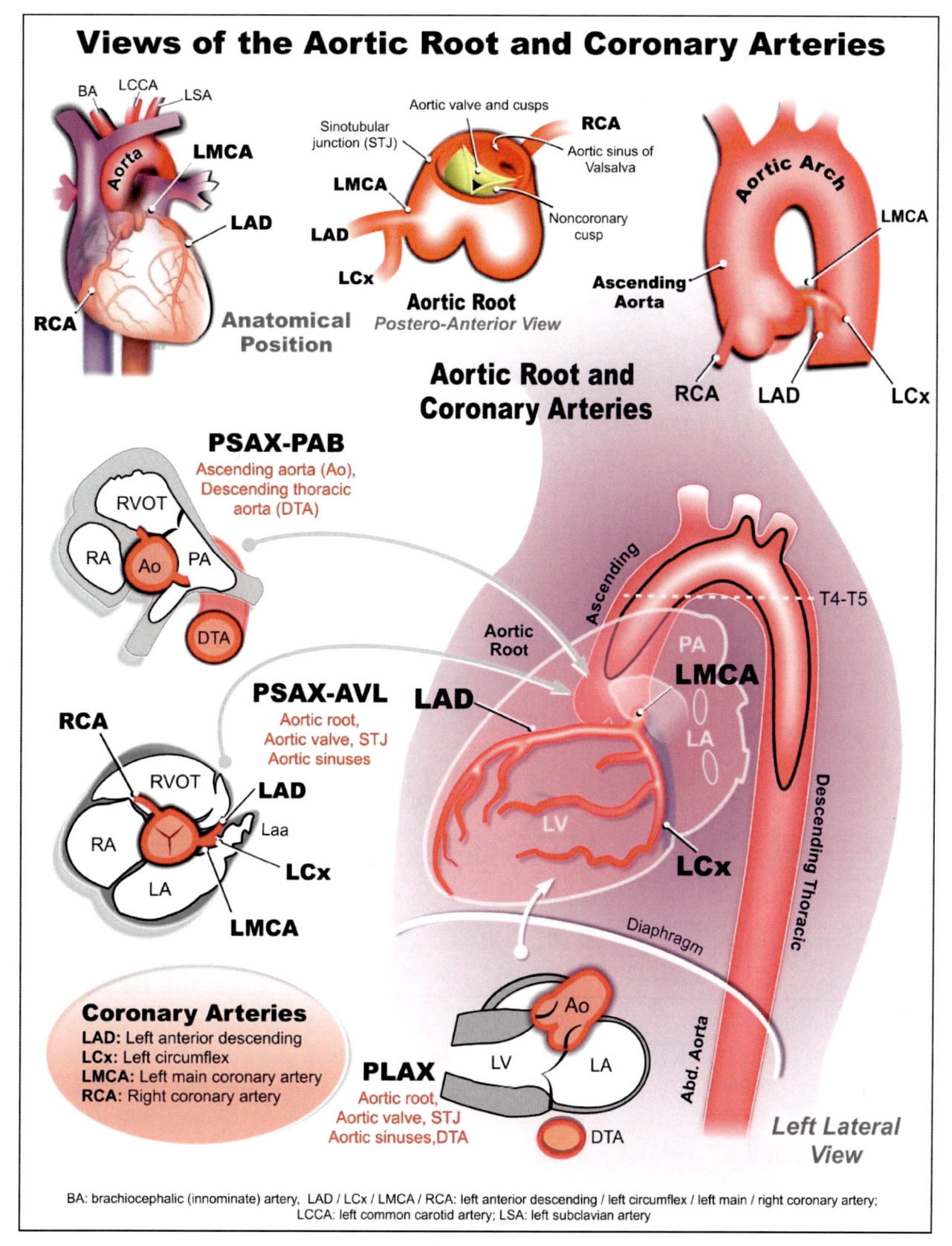

Fig 15. Echocardiographic views of the thoracic aorta, with focus on the aortic valve, and coronary arteries. Note the left main coronary (LMCA) and right coronary (RCA) arteries arising from the aortic root ~4 o'clock and ~10 o'clock positions on the PSAX-AVL view. Compare with Figs. 1-17.

PSAX-Aortic Valve Level and Coronary Arteries

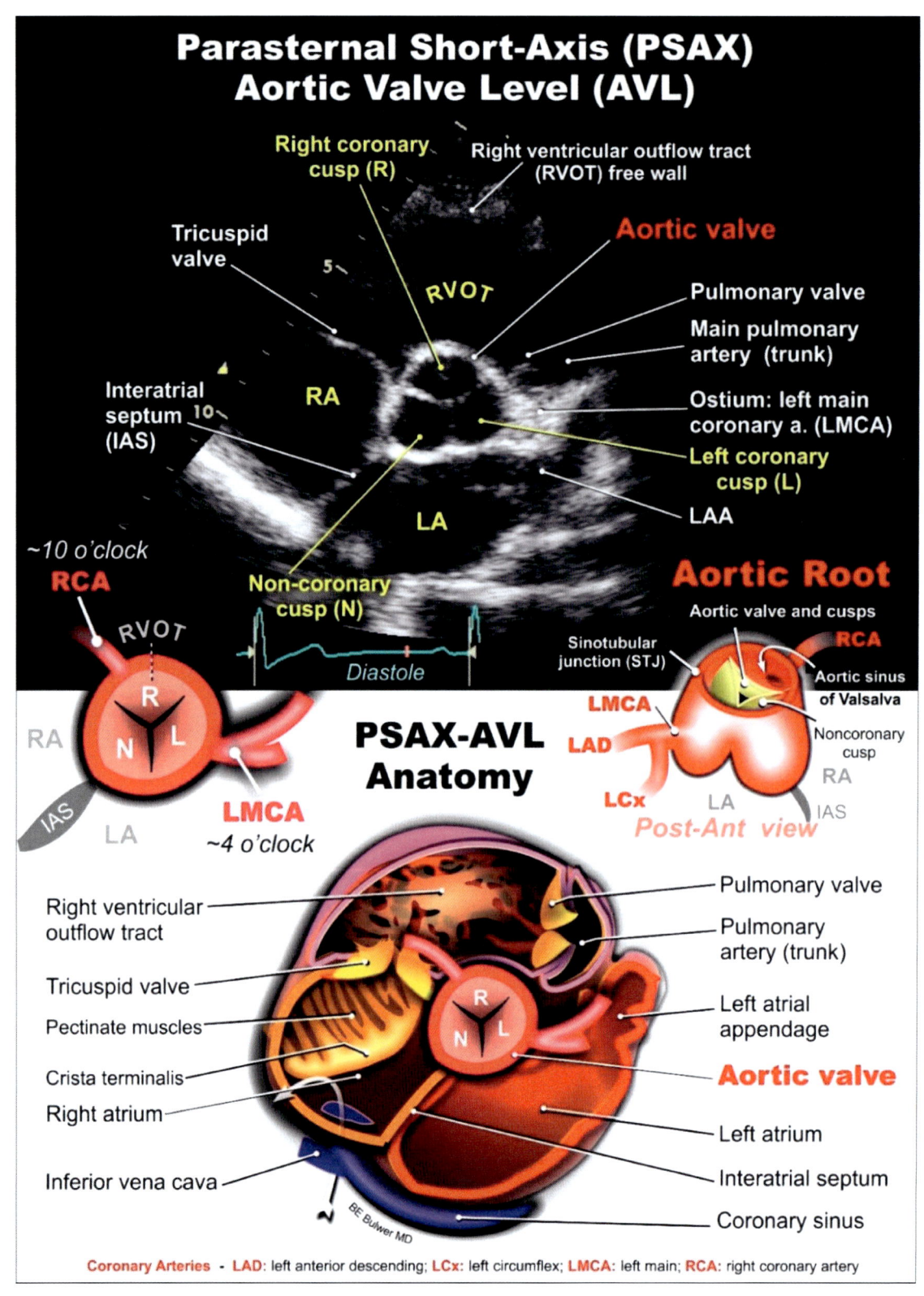

Fig 16. Parasternal short-axis view-aortic valve level (PSAX-AVL) and corresponding cross-sectional anatomy. Note the origins of the right (RCA) and left main coronary arteries (LMCA) emerging from the right and left coronary sinuses of Valsalva at ~10 o'clock and ~4 o'clock positions, respectively. The proximal portions of the RCA and LMCA are often best visualized just superiorly, at the level of the pulmonary artery bifurcation (see Fig. 14).

Coronary Artery Territories

PSAX Scan Planes and Corresponding Anatomy

Parasternal Short-Axis (PSAX) Scan Planes and Anatomy

PSAX Family of Scan Planes

PSAX-AVL Scan Plane

Anatomical Views

PSAX: Aortic Valve Level (AVL)

Labels: SVC, Aorta, RVOT, TV, RA, IVC, LAA, Aortic valve (AV), LA, Coronary sinus

A. PSAX Anatomy: Aortic Valve Level

- RVOT
- tricuspid valve (TV): septal leaflet
- antero-lateral leaflet (TV)
- pectinate muscles with crista terminalis
- noncoronary cusp (AV)
- right atrium (RA)
- inferior vena cava (IVC) with valve (Eustachian)
- right ventricular outflow tract (RVOT)
- pulmonary valve
- main pulmonary artery
- left atrial appendage (LAA)
- right coronary cusp (AV)
- left coronary cusp (AV)
- left atrium (LA)
- interatrial septum
- coronary sinus

B. PSAX Anatomy: Aortic Root Level

- aortic root
- right atrial appendage (RAA)
- noncoronary cusp (AV)
- pectinate muscles with crista terminalis
- right atrium (RA)
- valve of the coronary sinus (Thebesian)
- inferior vena cava (IVC)
- main pulmonary artery
- left pulmonary artery
- left coronary cusp (AV)
- left main coronary artery (LMCA)
- left atrial appendage (LAA)
- left upper pulmonary vein (LUPV)
- left atrium (LA)
- interatrial septum
- coronary sinus

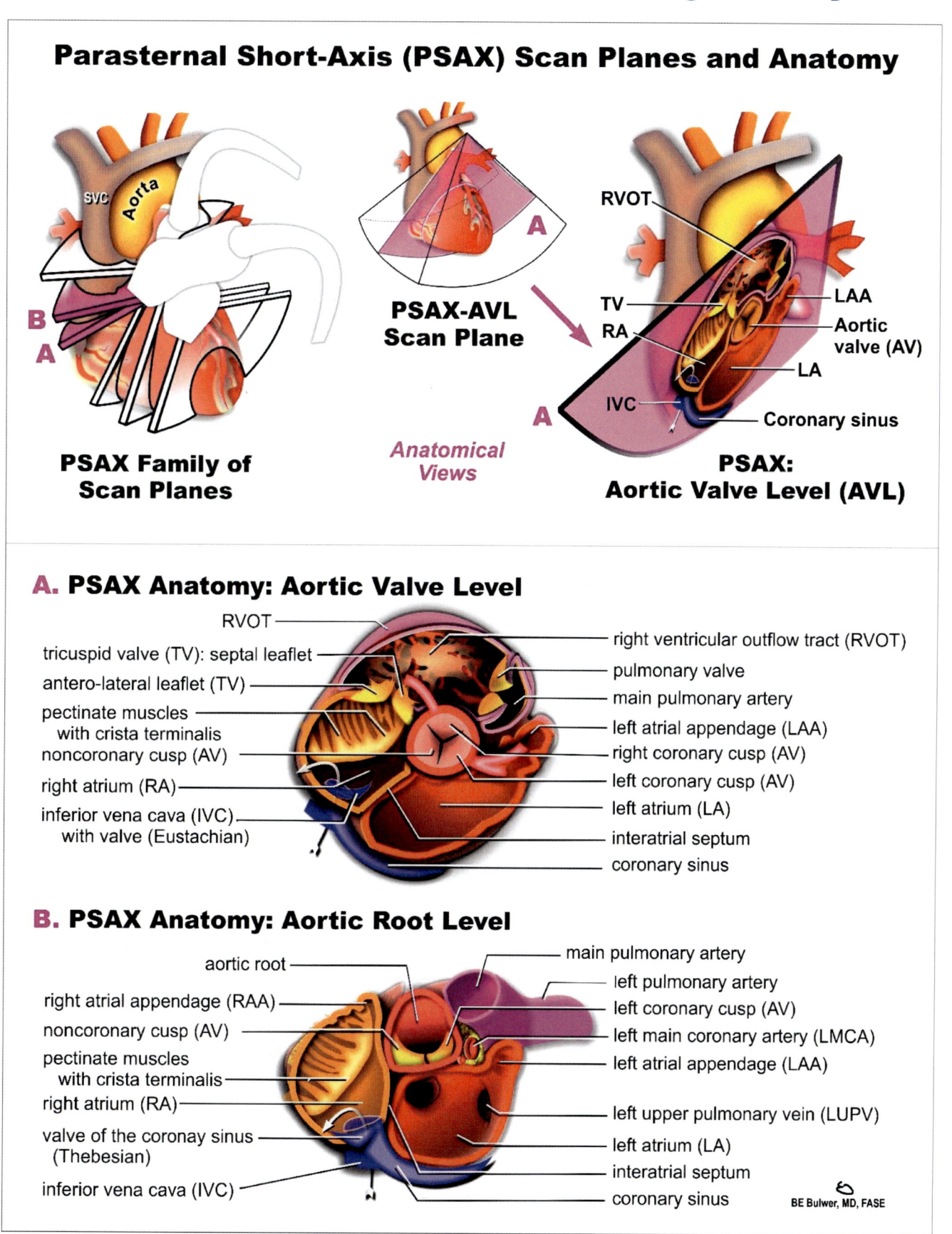

BE Bulwer, MD, FASE

Fig. 17. Anatomy of the parasternal short-axis view at the level of the aortic valve (PSAX-AVL). Compare with Figs. 12-18).

TEE of the Aortic Valve and Coronary Arteries

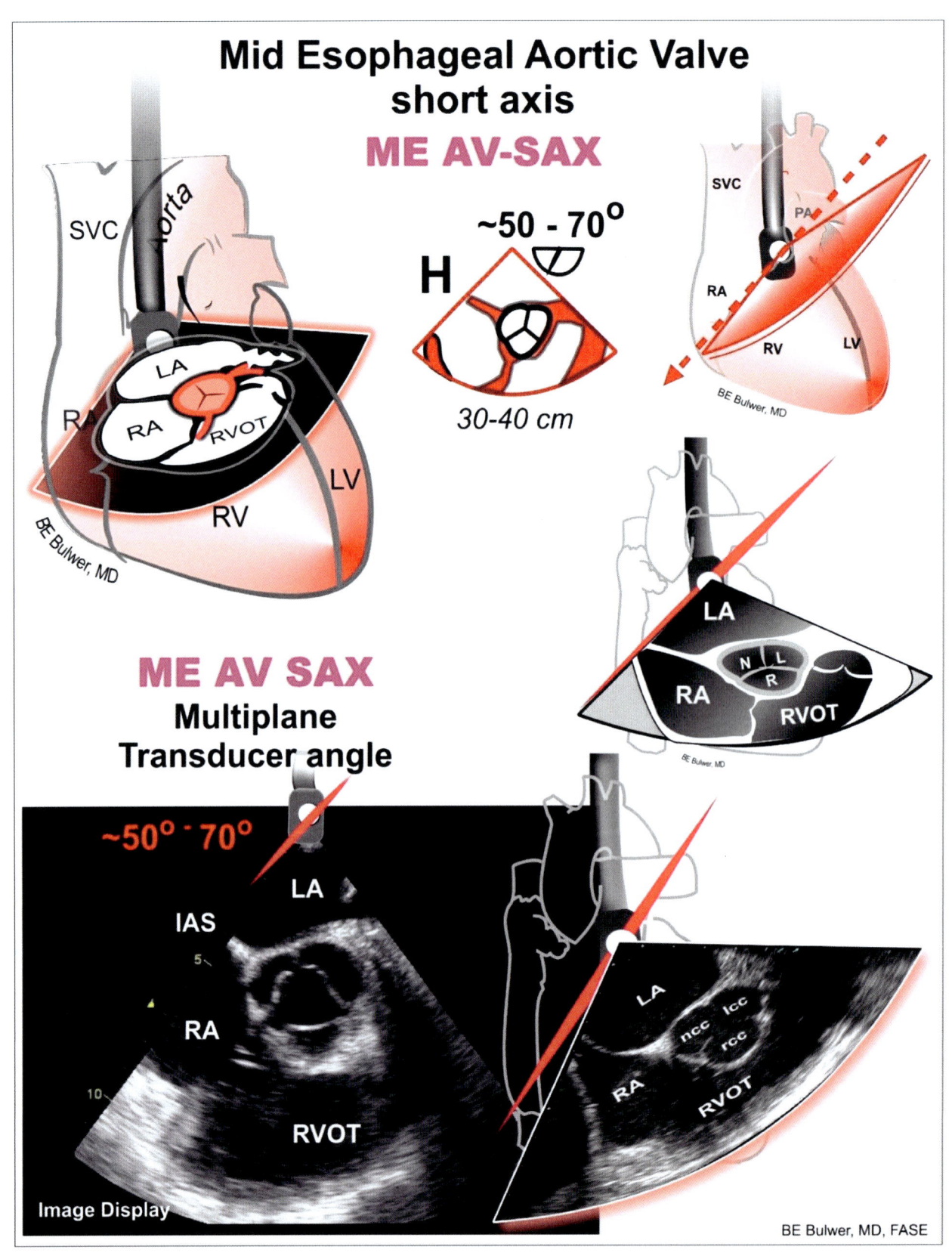

Fig. 18. Cross-sectional anatomy of the mid-esophageal-aortic valve short-axis (ME-AV-SAX) view on transesophageal echocardiography (TEE). Essentially, the same structures are imaged on the parasternal short-axis view-aortic valve level (PSAX-AVL) on transthoracic echocardiography (TTE). Compare with Figs. 12-17.

Coronary Artery Territories

PSAX View-Mitral Valve Level and Basal LV Segments

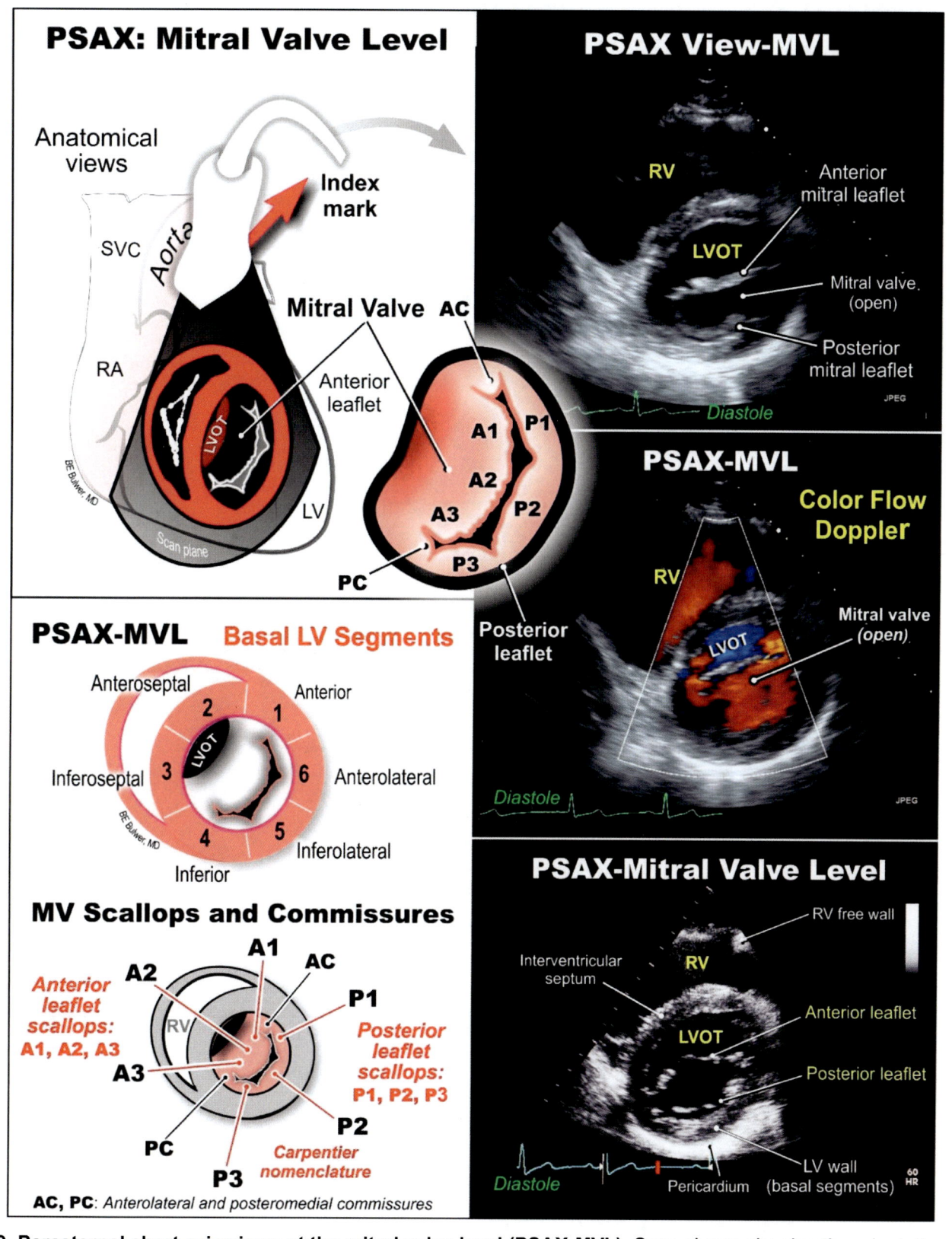

Fig. 19. Parasternal short axis views at the mitral valve level (PSAX-MVL). Scan planes showing the orientation of mitral leaflets and scallops *(upper and lower panels)*. Note the six basal segments of the left ventricle numbered 1 to 6. Note the coronary artery supply to these segments, which arises from both right and left coronary arteries as depicted in Figs. 21 (see Figs. 1-8).

PSAX Views-Mid LV and Apical LV Segments

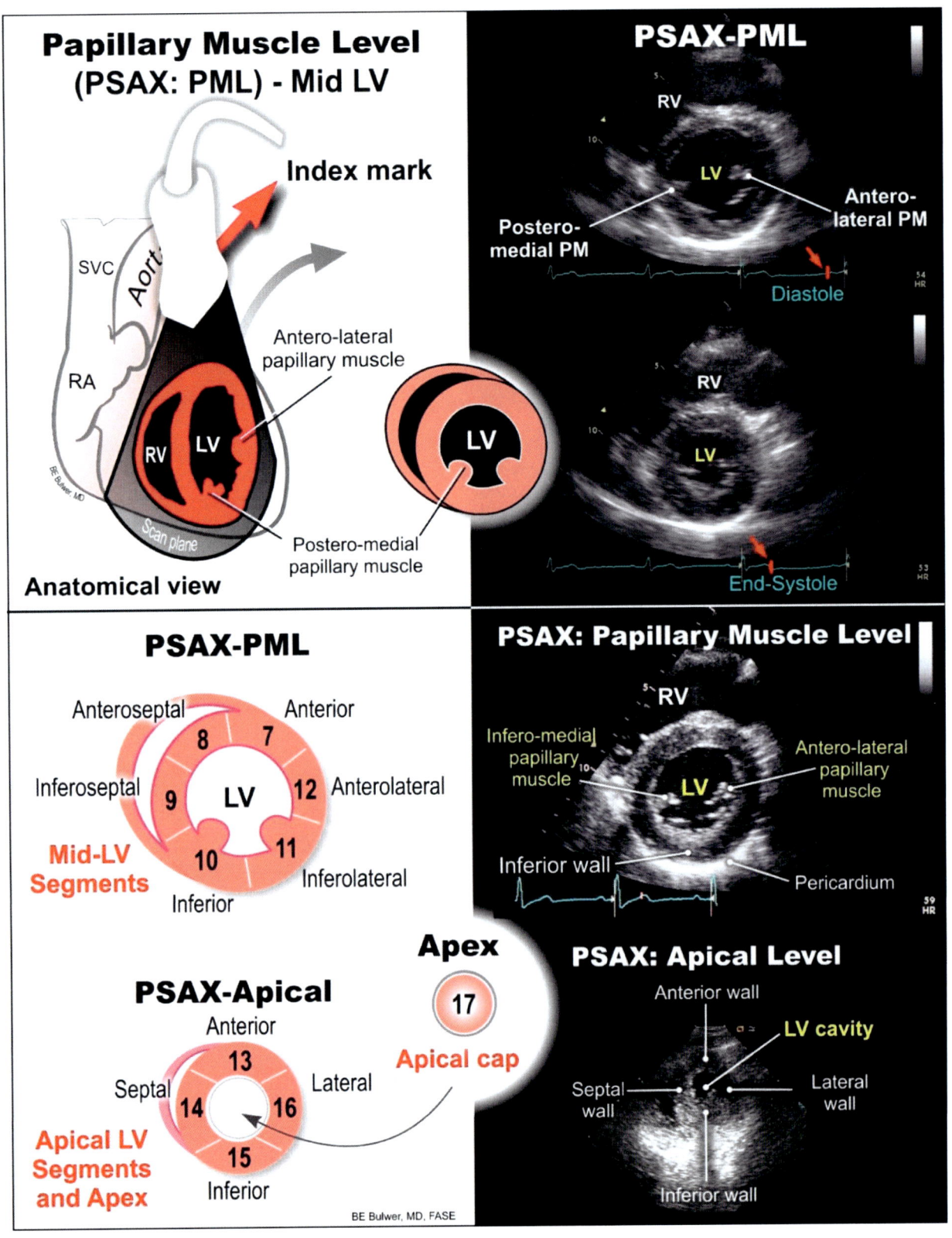

Fig 20. Parasternal short axis views at the mid-LV or papillary muscle level (PSAX-PML), at the LV apical level (PSAX-Apical), and at the LV apex or apical cap. Note scan planes depicting a pair of papillary muscles *(upper and lower panels)*. Note the six mid-LV segments numbered 7 to 12 and the four apical LV segments labeled 13-16, with the apical cap numbered 17. Note coronary artery supply to these segments, which arises from both right and left coronary arteries as depicted in Fig. 21 (see Figs. 1-8).

PSAX Views, LV Segments, and Coronary Artery Supply

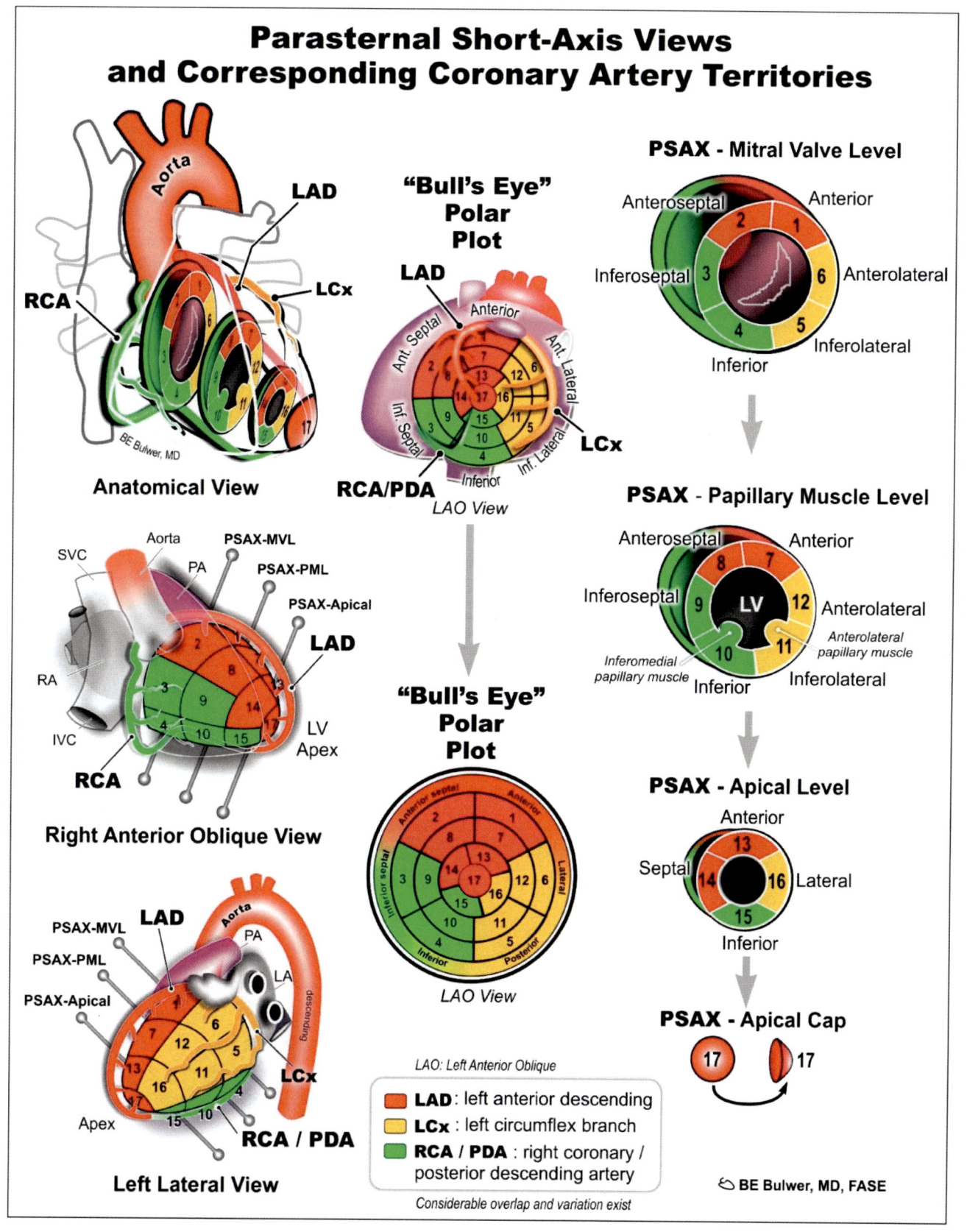

Fig 21. Parasternal short-axis (PSAX) views of the left ventricular walls—from the basal segments at the level of the mitral valve to the LV apex—are typically supplied by the major coronary arteries shown. Compare with Figs. 1-8, 32-34.

A4C View, LV Walls, and Coronary Artery Supply

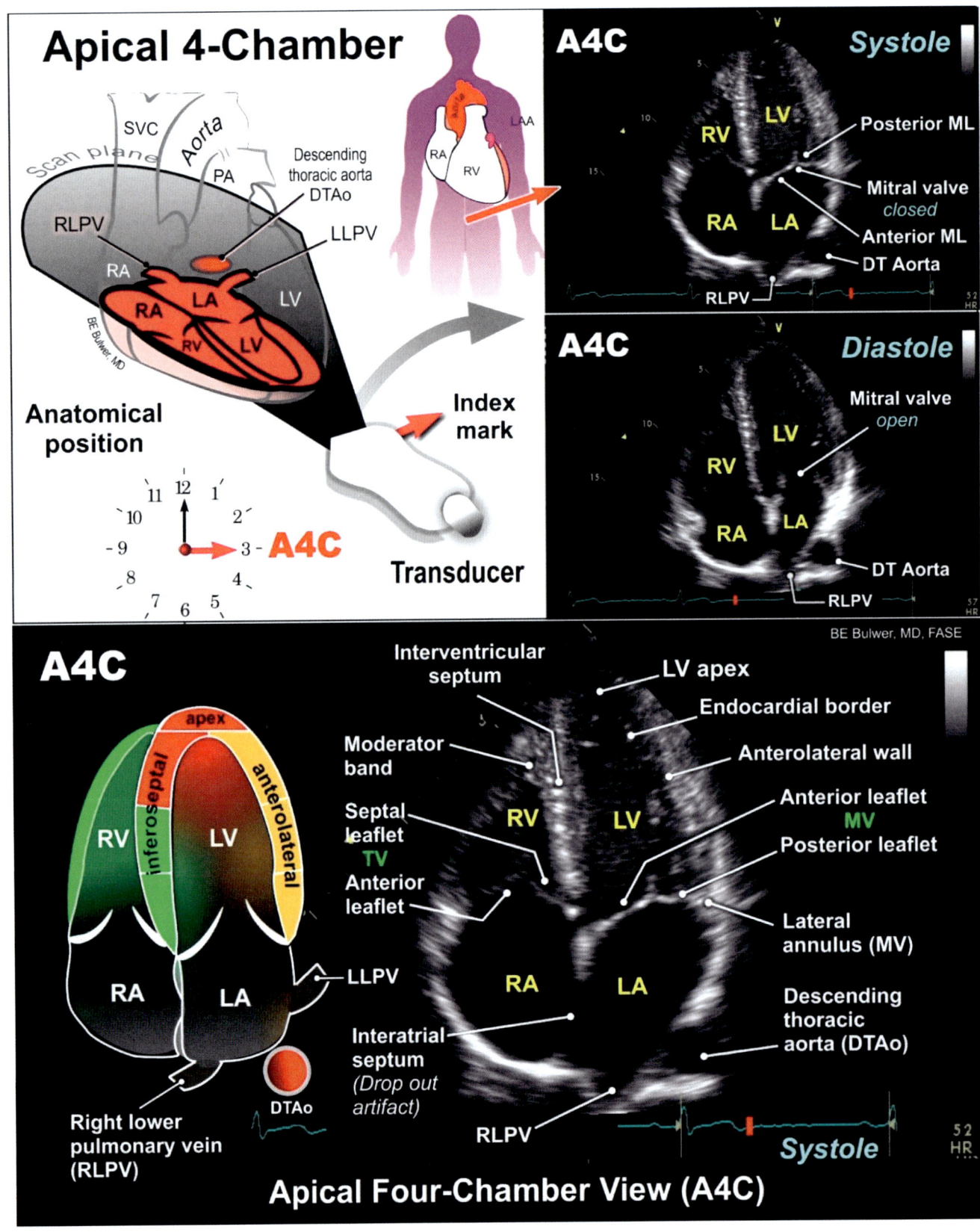

Fig 10. Apical four-chamber (A4C) views showing the left ventricular walls—the inferoseptal and anterolateral walls, and the LV apex. The corresponding LV segments are supplied by the left anterior descending (LAD), left circumflex (LCx), and right coronary (RCA) arteries as shown in Fig. 23. Compare with Figs. 1-8, 32-34.

Coronary Artery Territories

A4C View, LV Segments, and Coronary Artery Supply

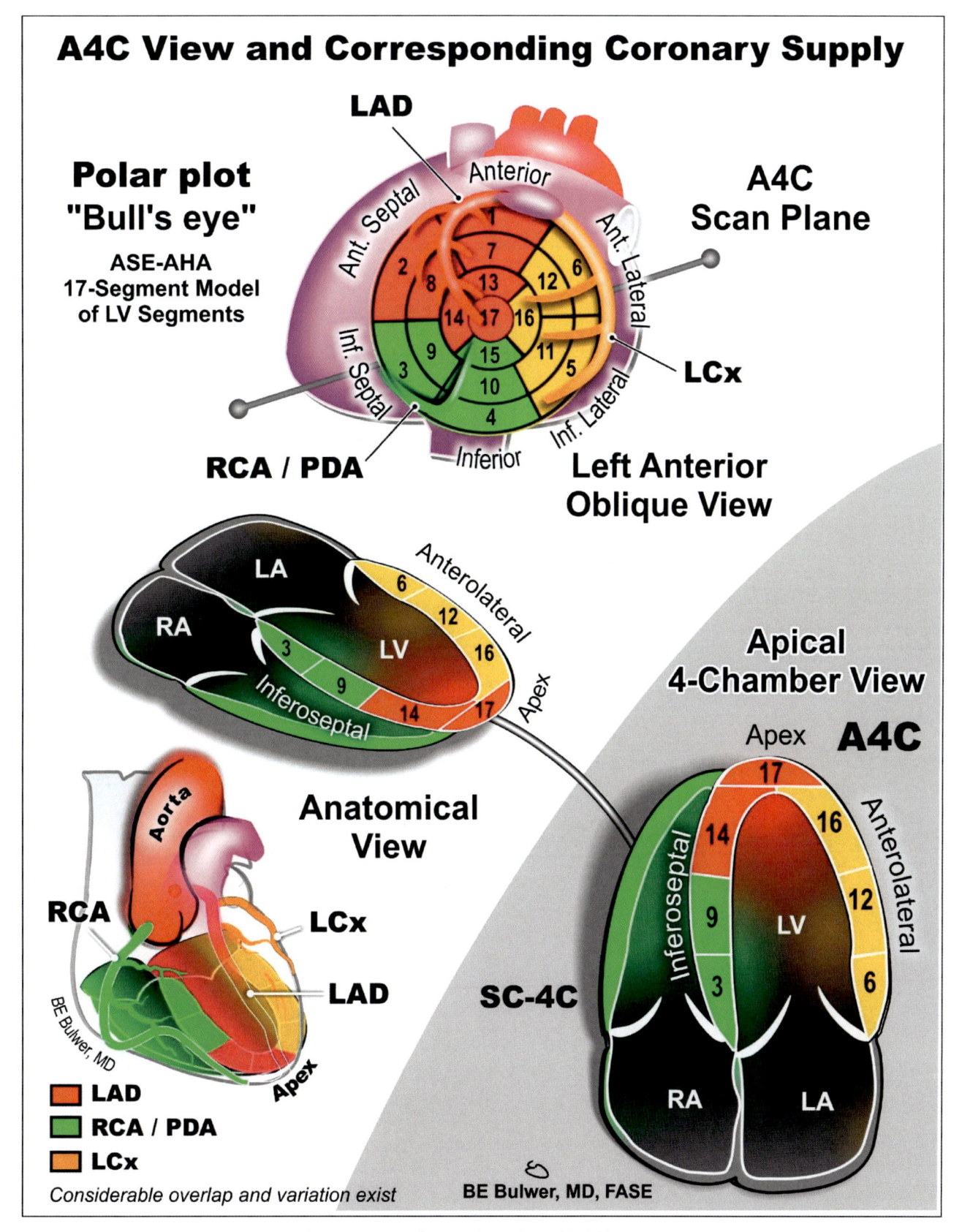

Fig 23. Panoramic perspectives of the apical four-chamber (A4C) view, the left ventricular (LV) walls and corresponding segments, and their coronary artery supply.

A2C View, LV Walls, and Coronary Artery Supply

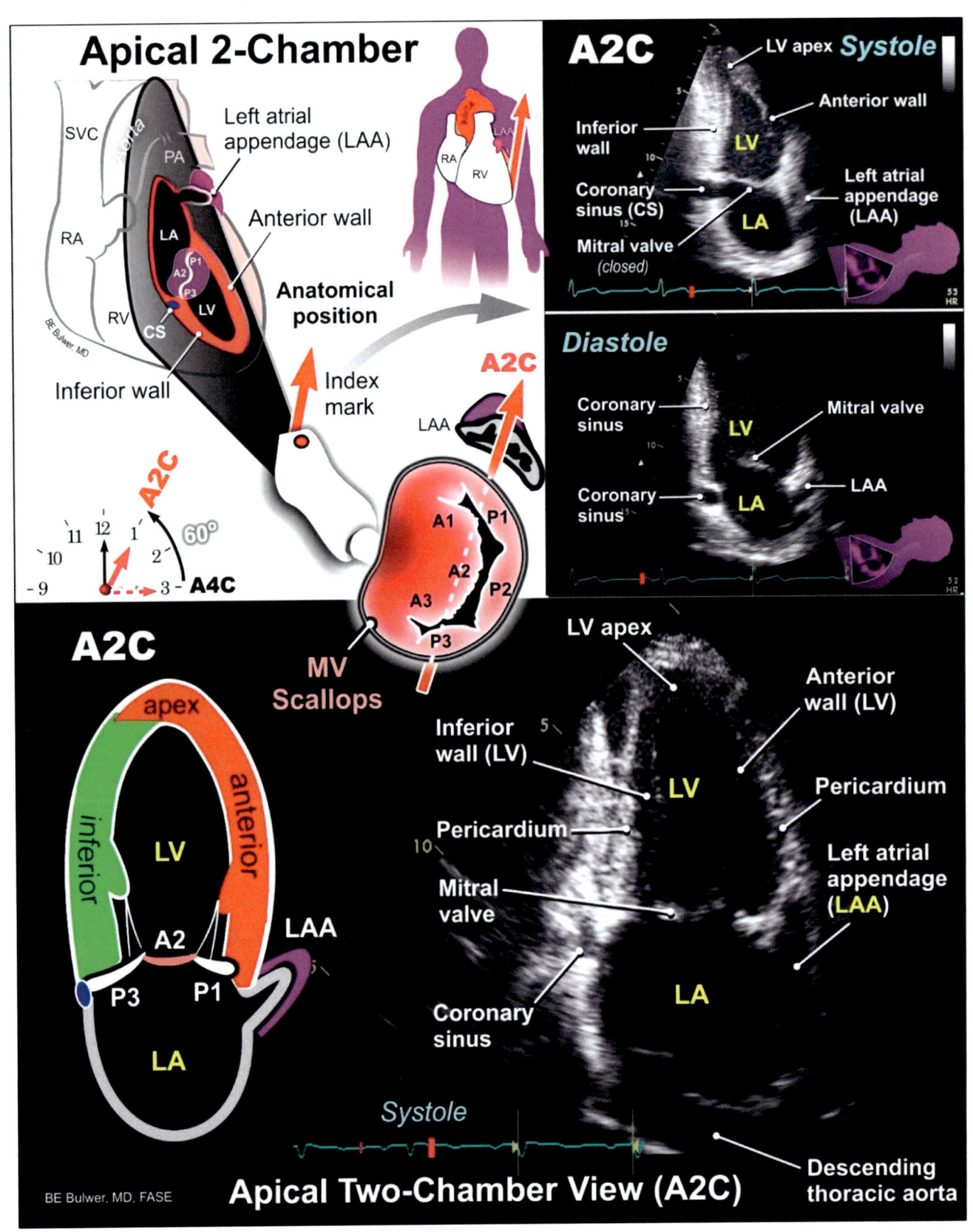

Fig 24. Apical two-chamber (A2C) view. The left ventricular walls seen on the A2C view—the anterior and inferior walls, and the LV apex—are typically supplied by the left anterior descending (LAD), and the posterior descending branch of the right coronary (RCA) arteries as shown. Compare with Figs. 1-8, 25, 32-34.

Coronary Artery Territories

A2C View, LV Segments, and Coronary Artery Supply

Apical 2-Chamber View

Anatomical view

- **LAD**: left anterior descending artery
- **RCA / PDA**: right coronary-posterior desc.
- **LCx**: left circumflex artery

Considerable overlap and variation exist

A2C Plane (Vertical Long-axis Plane)

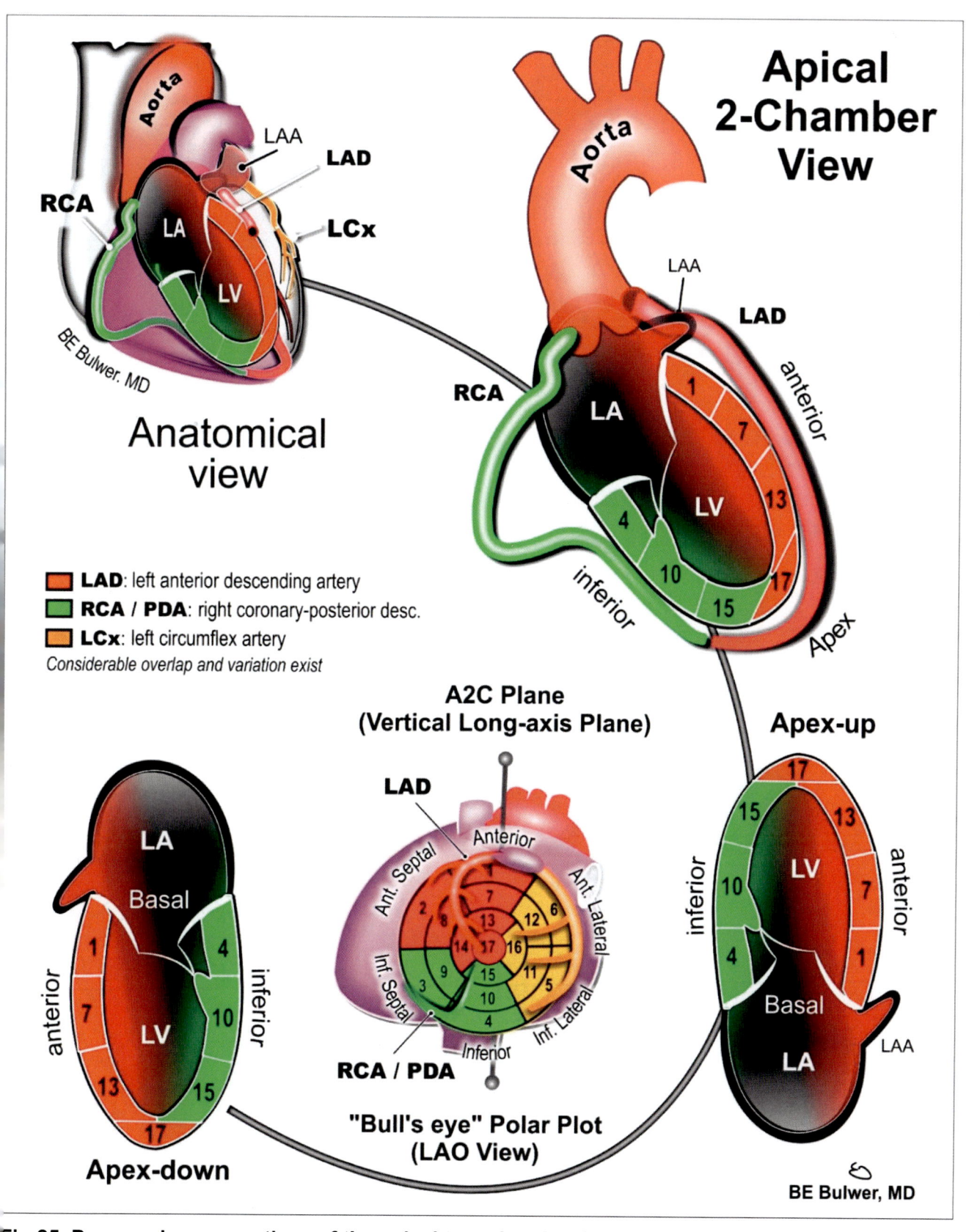

"Bull's eye" Polar Plot (LAO View)

Apex-up

Apex-down

Fig 25. Panoramic perspectives of the apical two-chamber (A2C) view, the left ventricular (LV) walls and corresponding segments, and their coronary artery supply.

A3C View, LV Walls, and Coronary Artery Supply

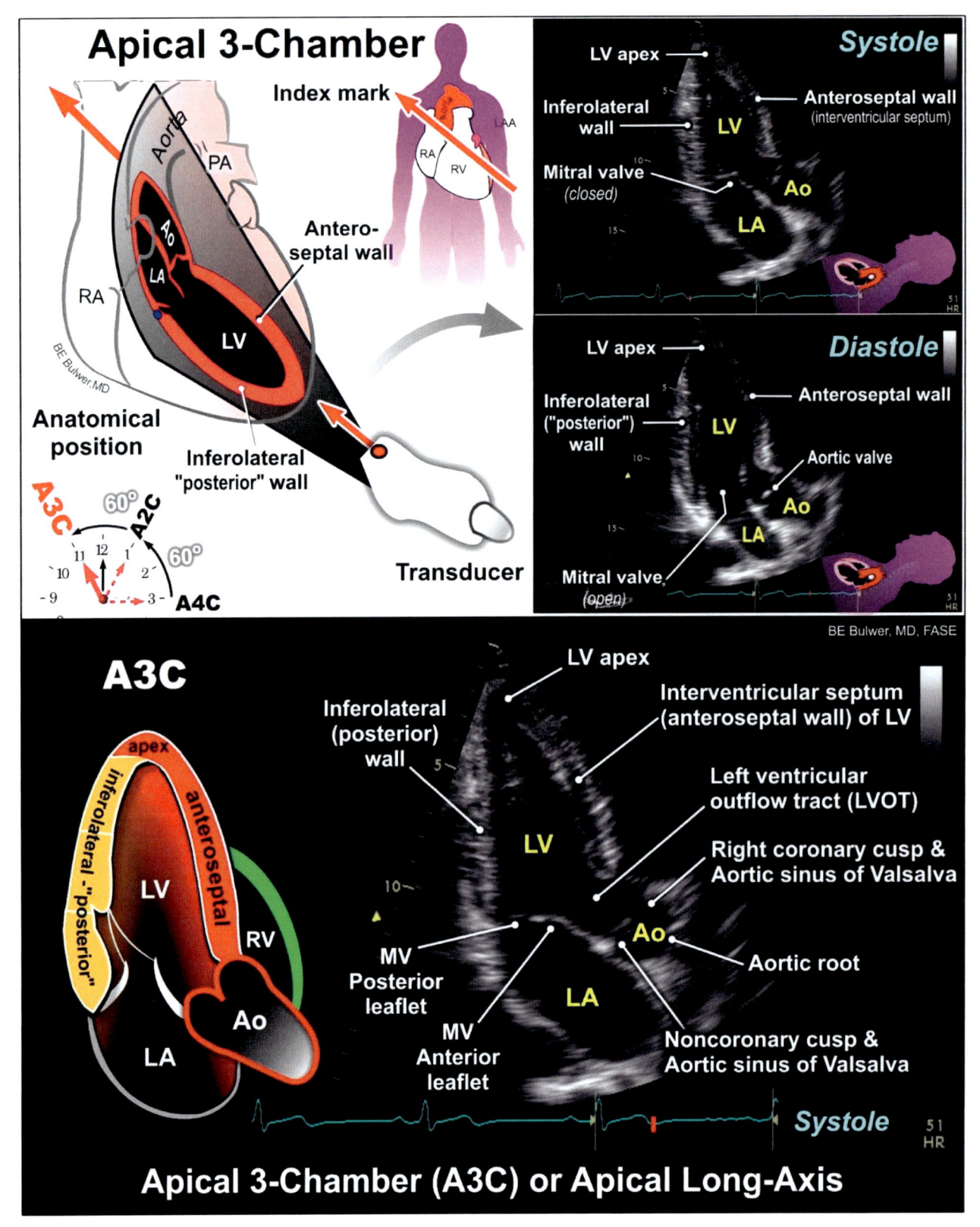

Fig 26. **Apical three-chamber (A3C) or apical long-axis (ALAX) view.** The LV walls seen on the A3C view—the anteroseptal wall (interventricular septum) and the inferolateral (posterior) wall—are typically supplied by the left anterior descending (LAD) and the left circumflex (LCx) coronary arteries. Compare with Figs. 1-11, 32-34

Coronary Artery Territories

A3C View, LV Segments, and Coronary Artery Supply

Apical Long-axis (A3C) Views

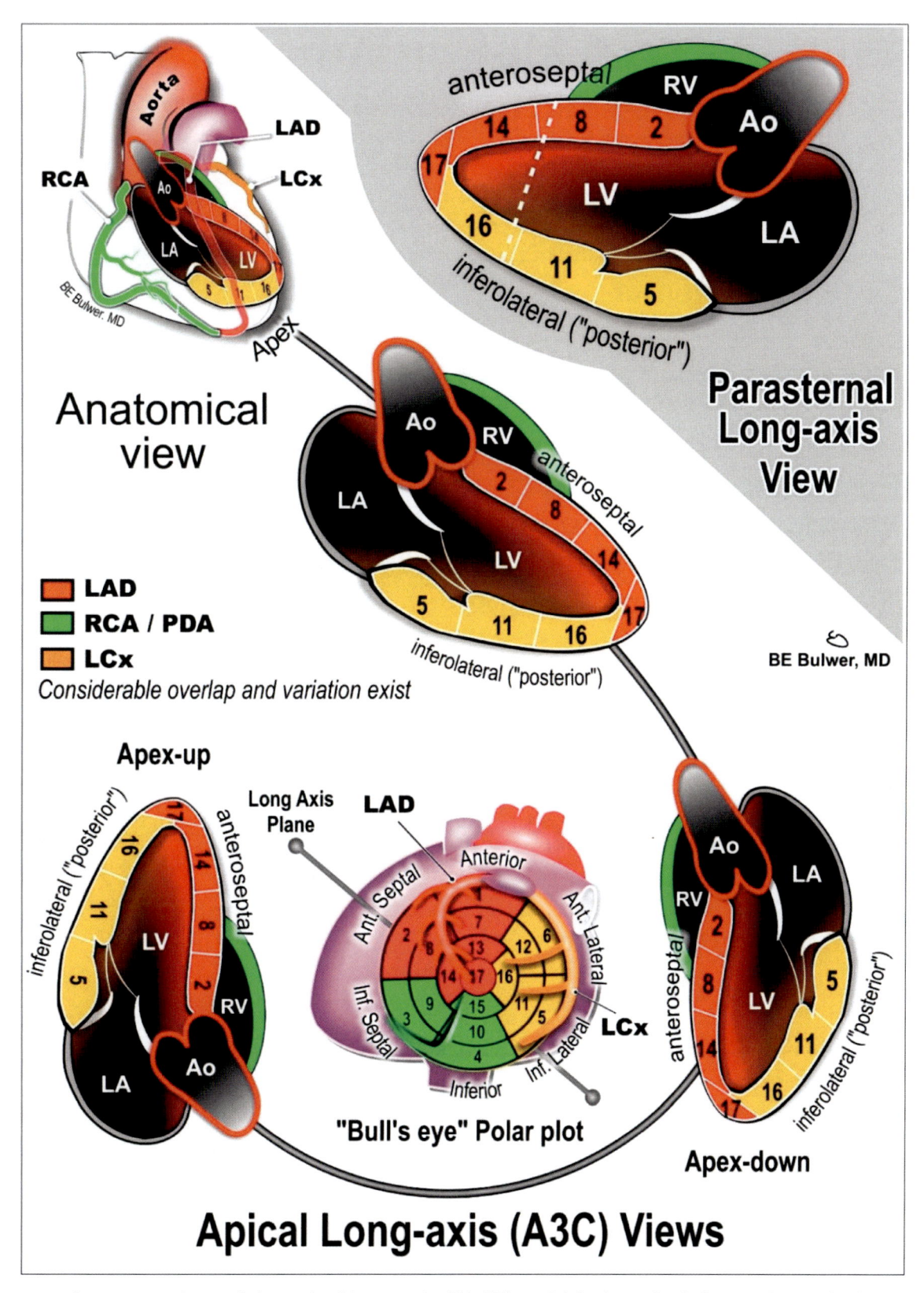

Fig 27. Panoramic perspectives of the apical long-axis (ALAX) or A3C view, the left ventricular (LV) walls and corresponding segments, and their coronary artery supply. The LV segments seen on the ALAX (A3C) view are also seen on the parasternal long-axis (PLAX) view. However, the ALAX view includes the LV apical segments, unlike the PLAX view. Compare with Figs. 1-8, 10, 11, 56-58).

Wall Motion Abnormalities: Ischemic vs. Nonischemic

Regional Wall Motion Abnormalities
Ischemic vs. Non-Ischemic

Inschemic - Coronary Artery Disease
- Acute Ischemia
- Chronic Ischemia

Conduction System Abnormalities
- Left bundle branch block (LBBB)
- Premature ventricular contractions (PAC)
- Ventricular preexcitation (Wolf Parkinson White, WPW)
- Ventricular pacing

Ventricular Interdependence
- Right ventricular (RV) pressure overload
- Right ventricular (RV) volume overload
- Constrictive Pericarditis

Miscellaneous
- Post cardiac surgery
- External compression (pseudodyskinesis)
- Pregnancy
- Hiatus hernia
- Ascites
- Relaxation abnormalities: early, late
- Congenital absence of the pericardium

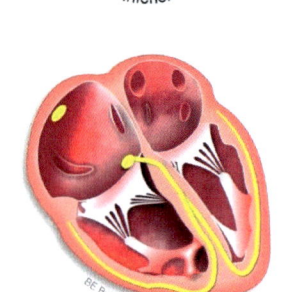

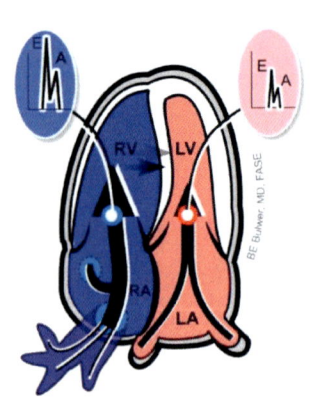

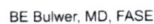

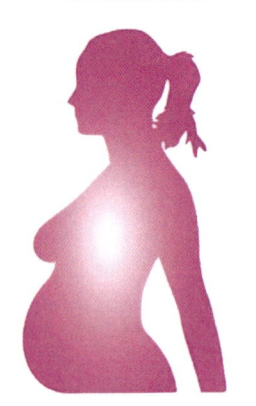

Fig. 28. Impaired movement and contractile function of the left ventricular walls, or wall motion abnormalities (WMA), can be secondary to ischemic and non-ischemic causes. Acute and chronic coronary ischemia is a leading cause of regional wall motion abnormalities (RWMA), which can be semi-quantitatively assessed by echocardiography (Figs. 29-75).

Ischemic Cascade: Utility of Echocardiography

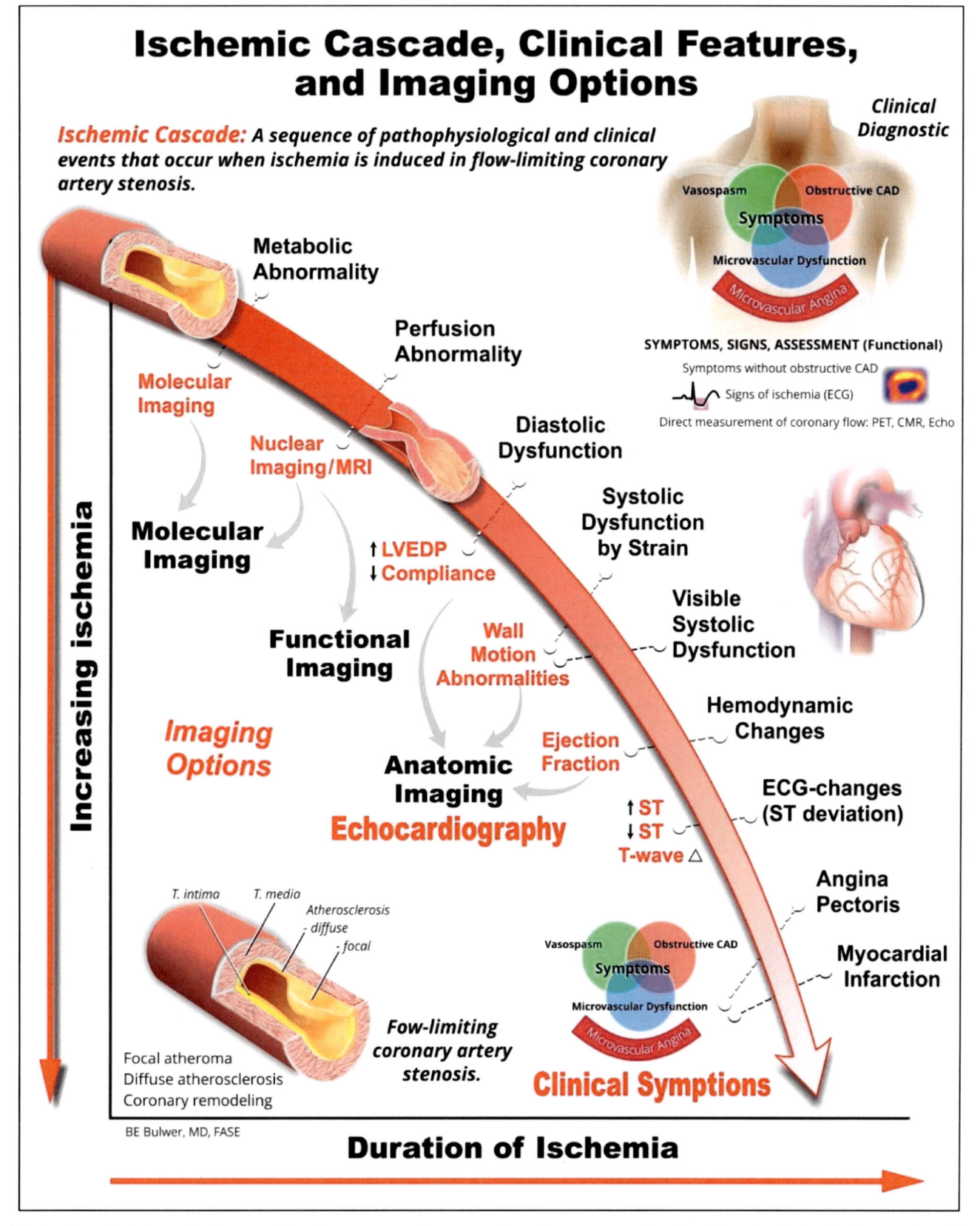

Fig 29. Ischemic injury to the ventricular myocardium can lead to a cascade of pathophysiological events called the ischemic cascade. Echocardiography is used to assess impaired systolic and diastolic function due to coronary ischemia, including regional wall motion abnormalities (RWMA). See Figs. 30-79.

Coronary Microvasculature and Clinical Correlates I

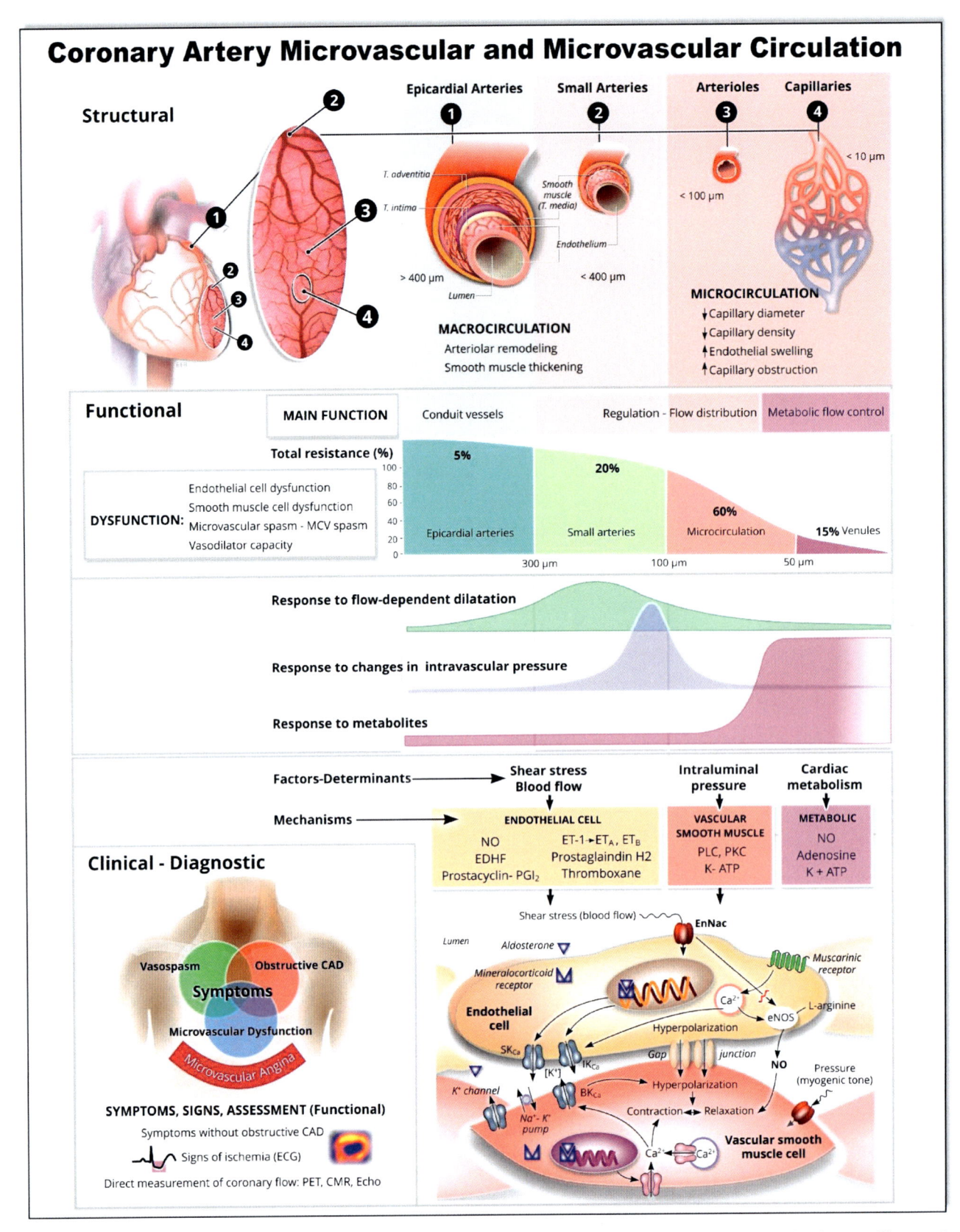

Fig 31. **The coronary arterial supply to the myocardium consists of network of progressively smaller and functionally distinct regions within the coronary tree, starting with the large epicardial arteries, to pre-arterioles, intramural arterioles, and the capillary bed.** The epicardial arteries are primarily conduits, compared to the pre-arterioles and arterioles which dynamically regulate and distribute blood flow to myocardial tissues.

Coronary Microvasculature and Clinical Correlates II

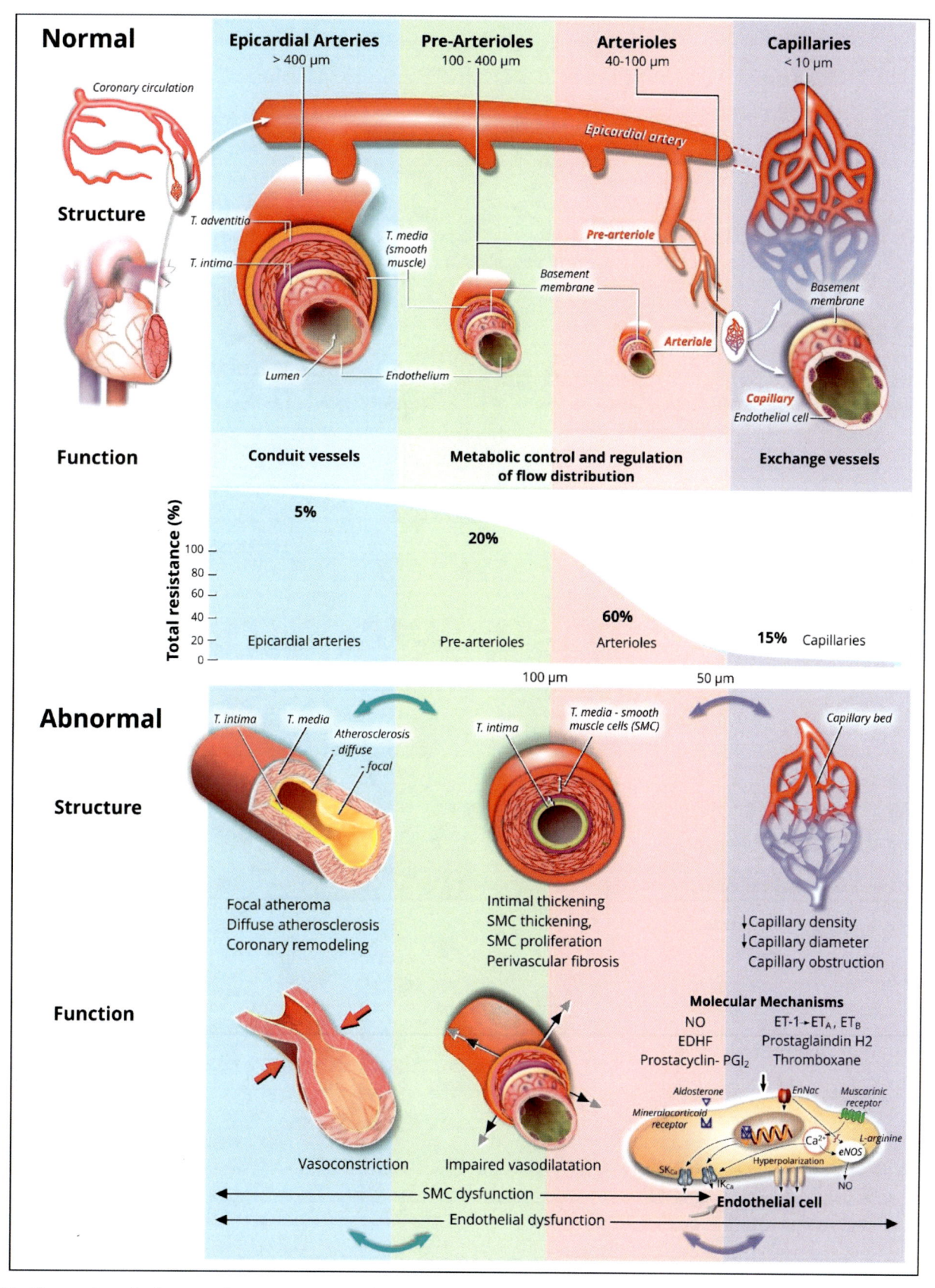

Fig 30. Normal and abnormal structure and function of the coronary arterial macrocirculation and microcirculation. EDHF = endothelium-derived hyperpolarizing factor; ET = endothelin; ET$_A$/ET$_B$ = endothelin receptors; NO = nitrous oxide; SMC = smooth muscle cell.

Coronary Ischemia and Wall Motion Assessment

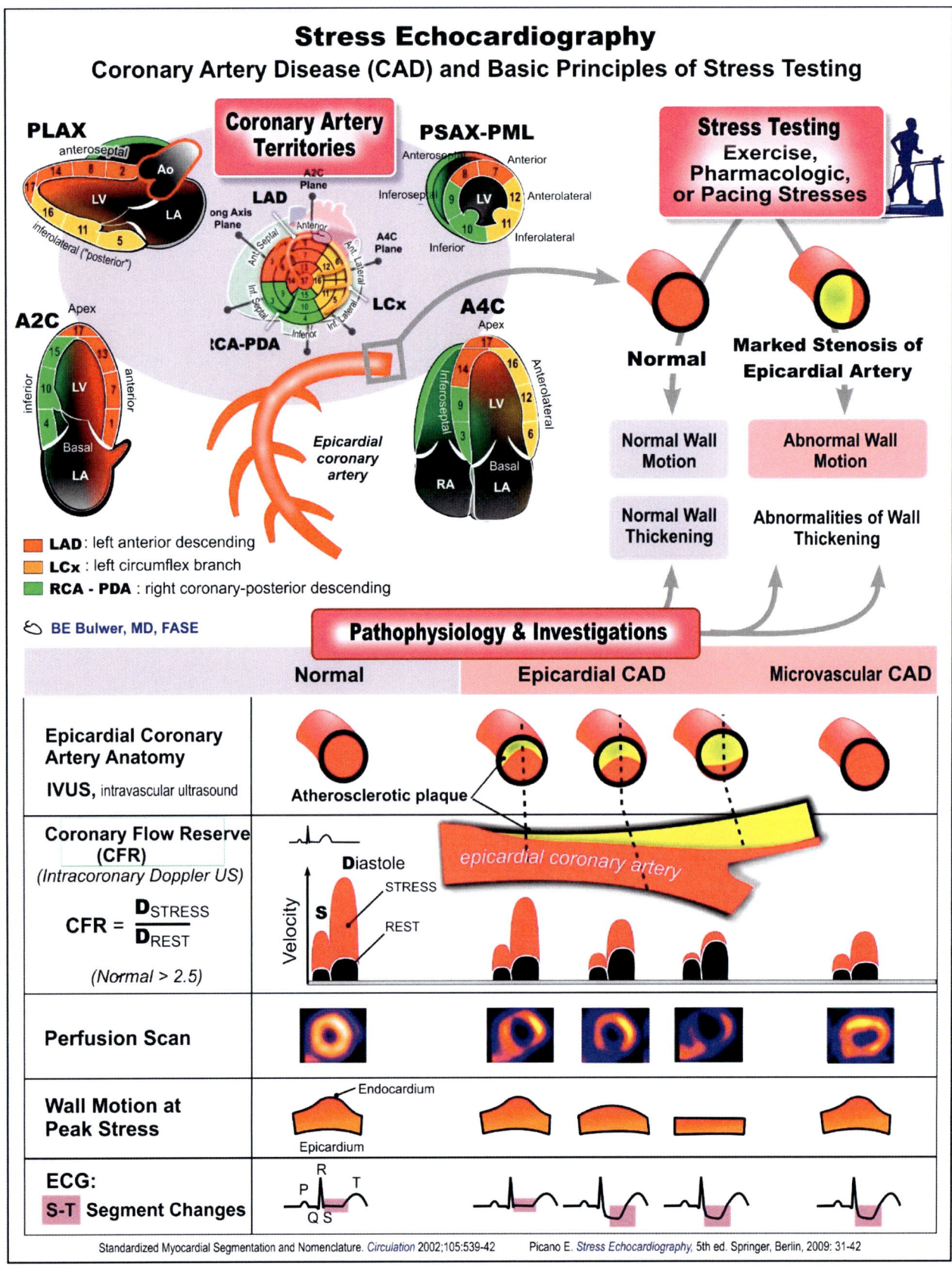

Fig. 32. Coronary artery disease and the basic principles of stress testing for coronary ischemia. Regional wall motion abnormalities (RWMA) observed on echocardiography are more sensitive and specific for coronary ischemia than ECG abnormalities—Compare with Fig. 29.

Wall Motion Assessment in Stress Echocardiography I

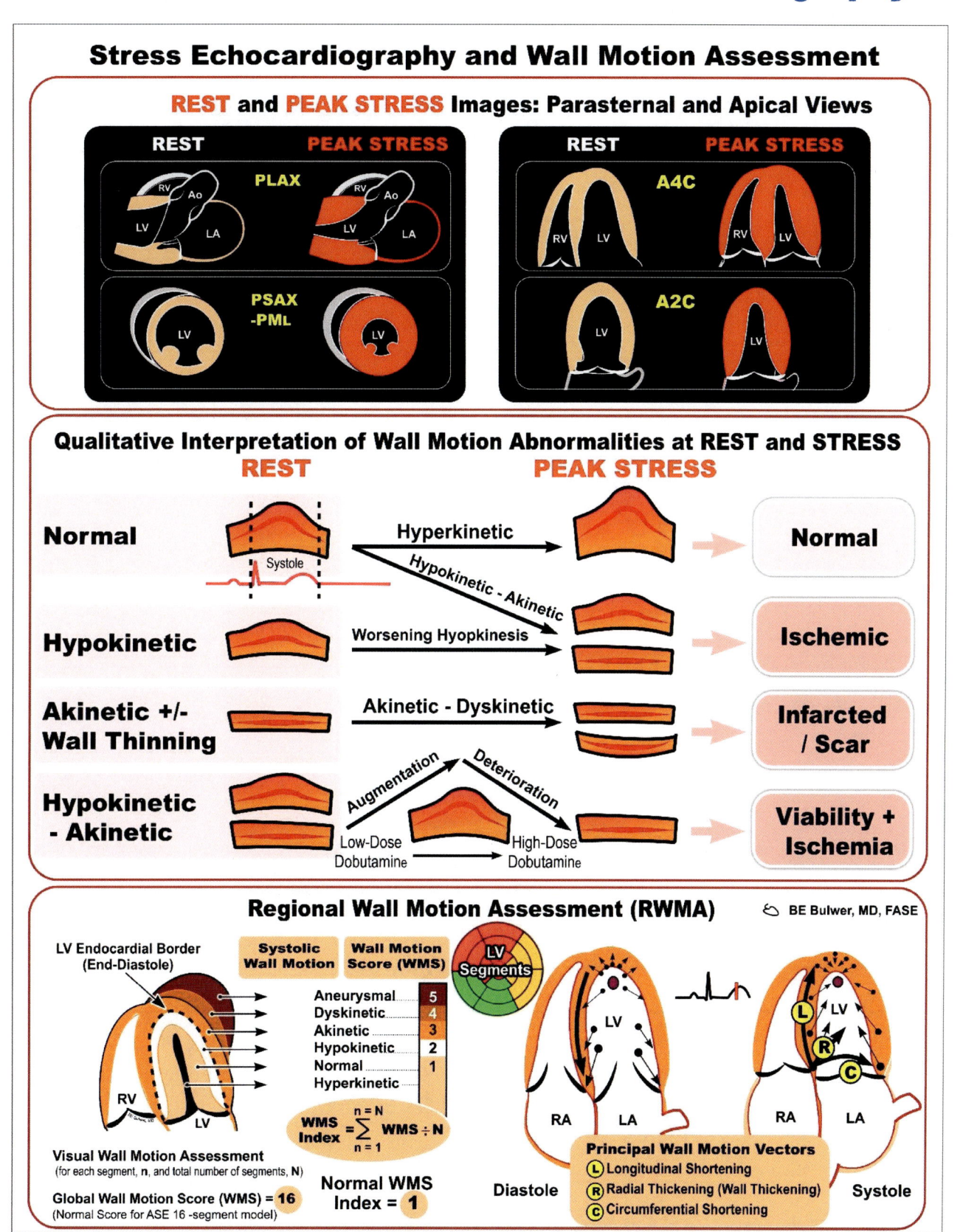

Fig. 33. The qualitative assessment *(middle panel)*, and in the semi-quantitative assessment *(lower panel)* of regional wall motion abnormalities in stress echocardiography (*see* Table Supplements to Fig. 83).

Wall Motion Assessment in Stress Echocardiography II

Stress Echocardiography Protocols

Bruce Exercise Stress Echo Protocol
Images: Rest and Immediate Post-Exercise (within 90 sec)

- Stage 1: 1.7 mph, Grade 10% (Slope) — 3 min
- Stage 2: 2.5 mph, Grade 12% — 3 min
- Stage 3: 3.4 mph, Grade 14% — 3 min
- Stage 4: 4.2 mph, Grade 16% — 3 min
- Stage 5: 5.0 mph, Grade 18% — 3 min
- Stage 6: 6.0 mph, Grade 20%

Bicycle Ergometer Stress Echo Protocol
Pedal Rate: 50 cycles / minute
Images: Rest, Intermediate, Peak Stress, and Recovery

- Stage 1: 25 Watts — 3 min
- Stage 2: 50 Watts — 3 min
- Stage 3: 75 Watts — 3 min
- Stage 4: 100 Watts — 3 min
- Stage 5: 125 Watts

Dobutamine Stress Echo Protocol for Ischemia
Images: Rest, Intermediate, Peak Stress, and Recovery

- Stage 1: 10 mcg/kg/min — 3 min
- Stage 2: 20 mcg/kg/min — 3 min
- Stage 3: 30 mcg/kg/min — 3 min
- Stage 4: 40 mcg/kg/min — 3 min

To achieve 85% of maximum age-predicted heart rate
Atropine: 0.25 to 0.5 mg boluses up to maximum dose of 2 mg

Dobutamine Stress Echo Protocol for Viability (Contractile Reserve)
Images: Rest, Low Dose and High Dose Dobutamine

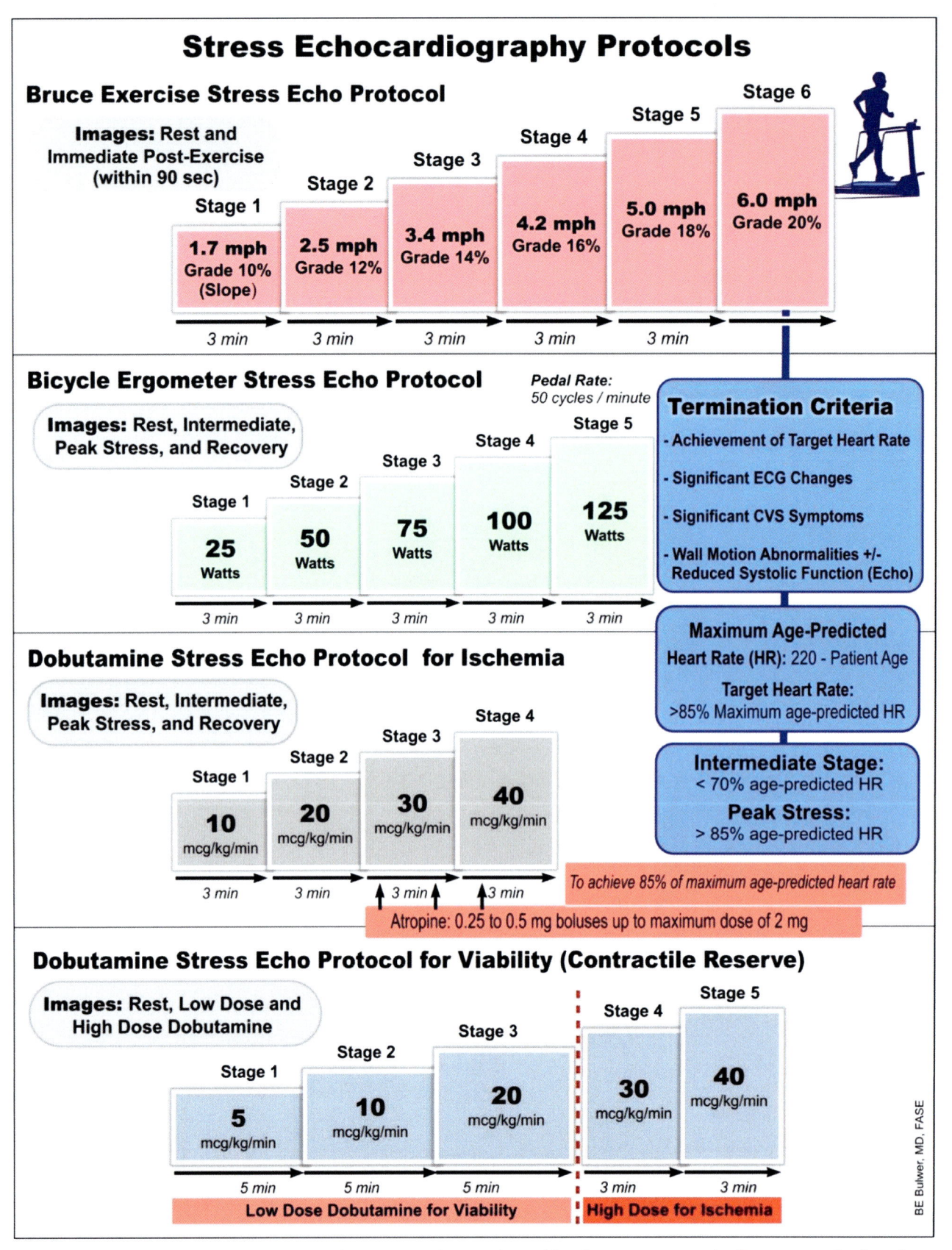

- Stage 1: 5 mcg/kg/min — 5 min
- Stage 2: 10 mcg/kg/min — 5 min
- Stage 3: 20 mcg/kg/min — 5 min
- Stage 4: 30 mcg/kg/min — 3 min
- Stage 5: 40 mcg/kg/min — 3 min

Low Dose Dobutamine for Viability | High Dose for Ischemia

Termination Criteria
- Achievement of Target Heart Rate
- Significant ECG Changes
- Significant CVS Symptoms
- Wall Motion Abnormalities +/- Reduced Systolic Function (Echo)

Maximum Age-Predicted Heart Rate (HR): 220 - Patient Age
Target Heart Rate: >85% Maximum age-predicted HR

Intermediate Stage: < 70% age-predicted HR
Peak Stress: > 85% age-predicted HR

Fig. 34. Various stress echocardiography protocols employed in the assessment of coronary ischemia. Echocardiographic assessment of regional wall motion abnormalities (RWMA) is performed during the various stages shown. Compare with Figs. 32, 33, and Table 1.

Stress Echocardiography: Utility and Indications

Table 1.

Echocardiography (Echo) Protocol		Utility	Indications / Comments
Exercise Stress Echo	Treadmill, Bicycle: supine or upright	Diagnostic	• Patients with abnormal baseline ECG or limited exercise tolerance • Non-specific ST-T-wave changes • Left bundle branch block • Left ventricular hypertrophy • Digoxin therapy • Wolf-Parkinson-White syndrome
		Prognostic	• Chronic Coronary Artery Disease • Post-myocardial Infarction
		Risk Stratification	• In heart failure: contractile reserve, mitral valve function, right ventricular function • Perioperative evaluation for non-cardiac surgery
Pharmacologic Stress Echo	Sympathomimetic amines e.g. Dobutamine Dobutamine (± atropine)	As for Exercise Stress Echocardiography (in patients unable to exercise)	• Indications as for exercise stress echo (when patients unable to exercise) • Myocardial viability assessment (for biphasic response) • Contractile reserve in patients with heart failure and low-gradient aortic stenosis
	Vasodilators e.g. Dypridamole, Adenosine	As for Exercise Stress Echocardiography (in patients unable to exercise)	• Less sensitivity than with sympathomimetic amines (used mainly outside the USA)
	Other: Ergonovine-Ergometrine, Enoximone	• Evaluation of vasospastic coronary artery disease	
Pacing Stress Echo	Atrial	• Diagnostic option for patients with known or suspected coronary artery disease (some centers)	
	Transesophageal atrial pacing		
Stress Echo with Doppler	Exercise treadmill, Supine bicycle	Low gradient aortic stenosis (with left ventricular dysfunction)	• Assessment of contractile reserve (Dobutamine stress)
		Heart failure; Assessment of systolic/diastolic dysfunction	• Mitral regurgitation and Trans-mitral Doppler indices using exercise or pharmacologic protocols.

Global Echo Measures of Myocardial Ischemia I

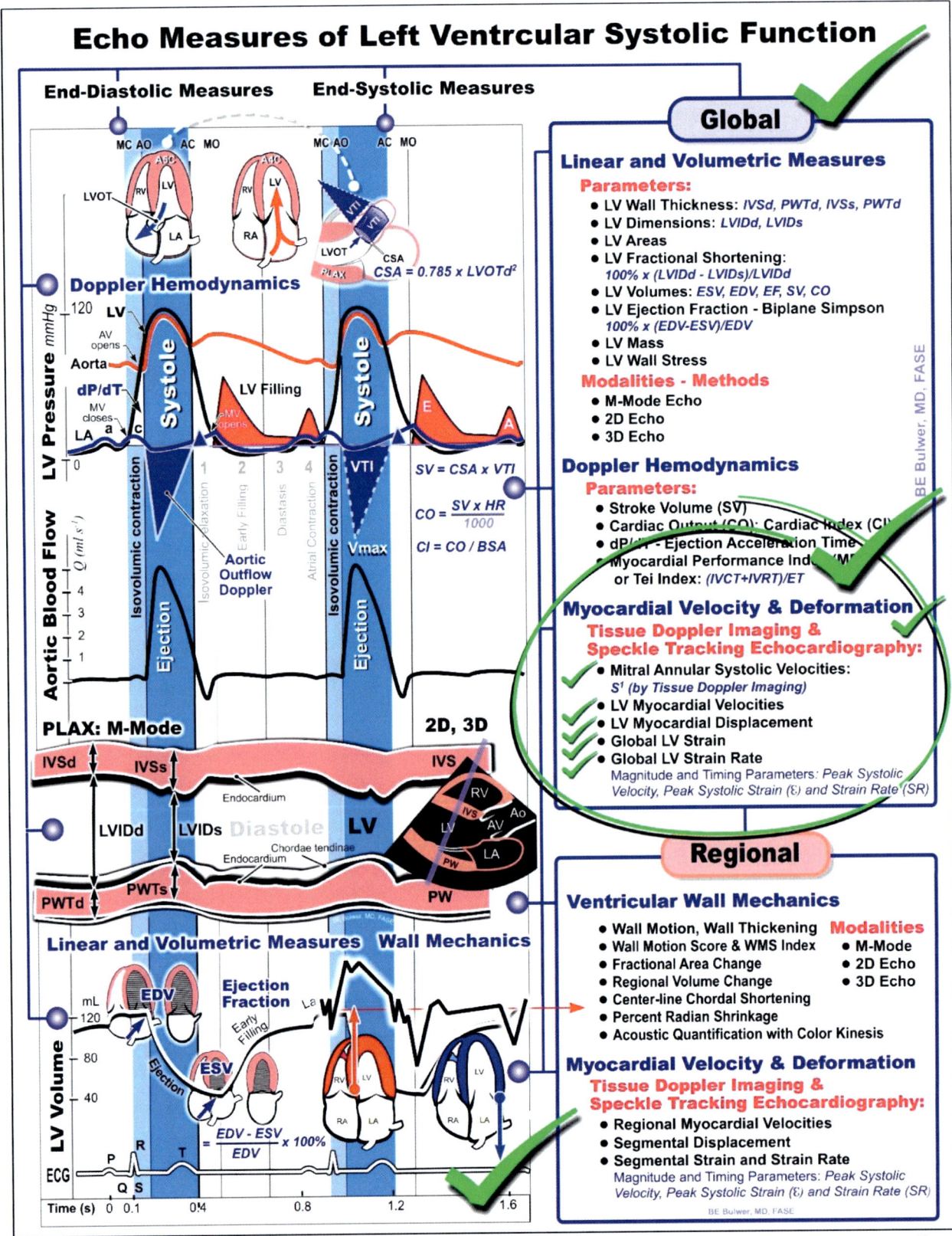

Fig 35. Summary of measures employed in the echocardiographic assessment of left ventricular systolic function. Myocardial ischemia leads to impairment of LV systolic function. Several parameters can be used to assess global and regional ventricular systolic function. Options for the global assessment of LV systolic function are highlighted here and in Fig. 36.

Global Echo Measures of Myocardial Ischemia II

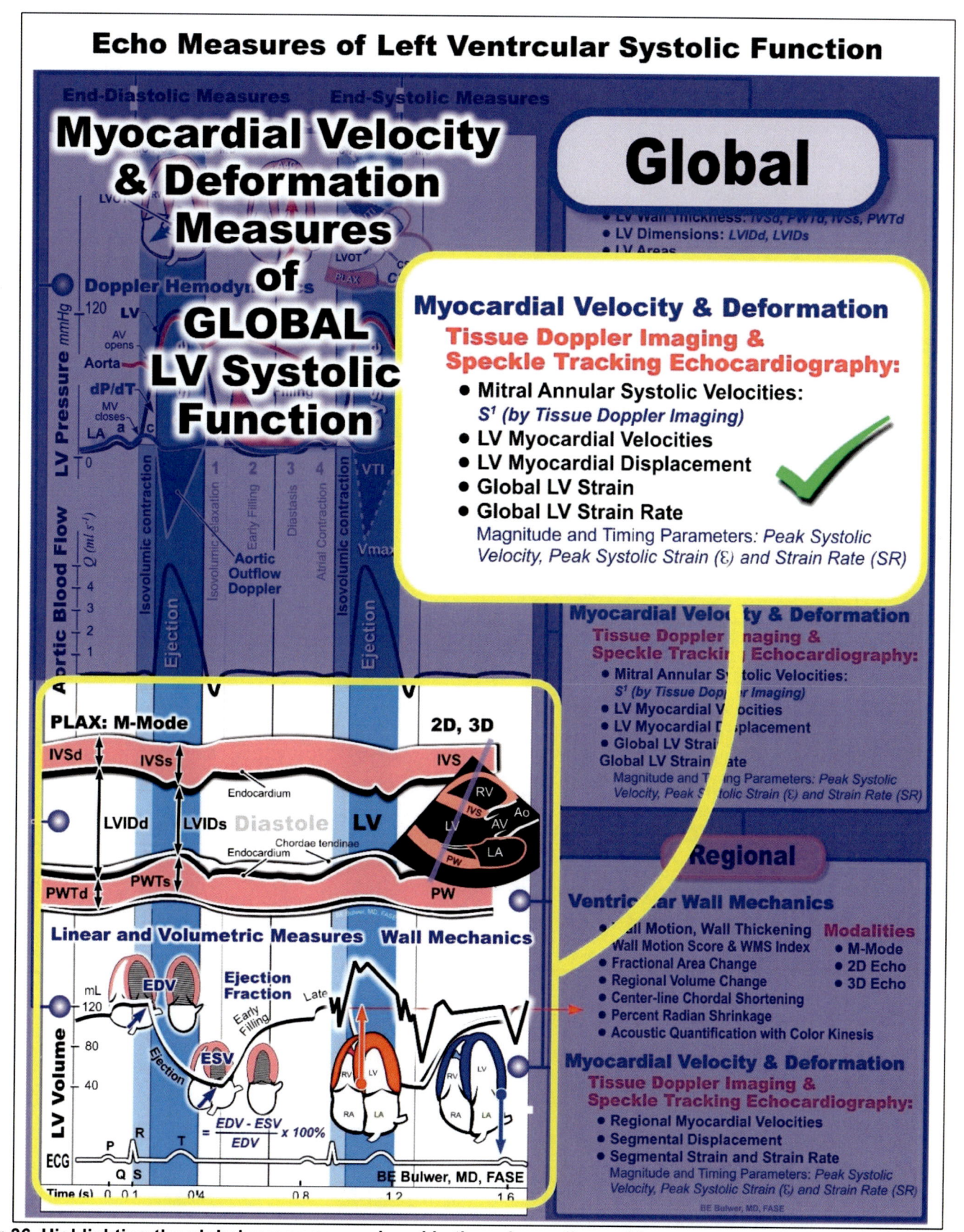

Fig 36. Highlighting the global measures employed in the echocardiographic assessment of left ventricular systolic function in patients with suspected or established coronary artery disease.

Deformation Parameters in Myocardial Ischemia I

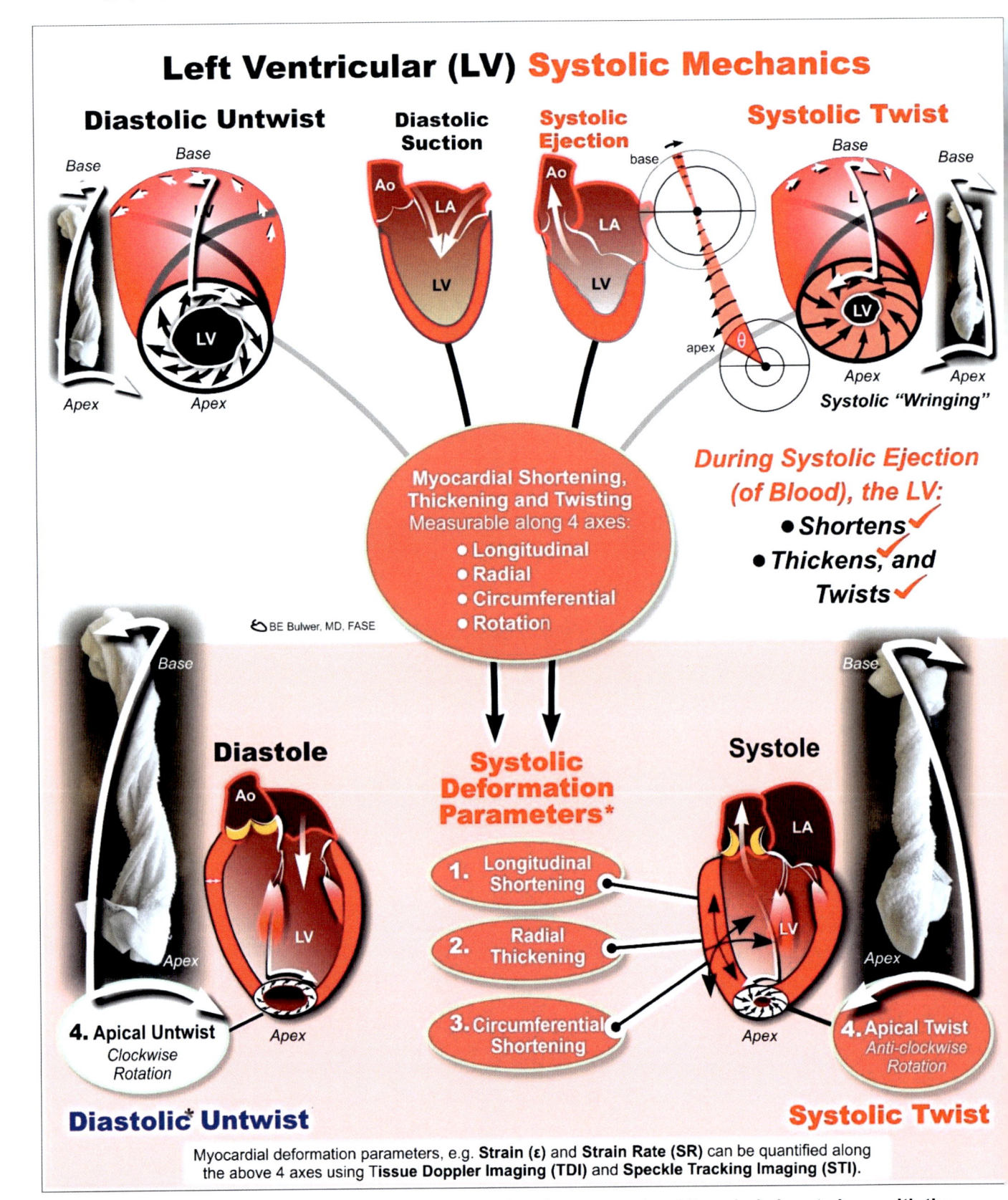

Fig. 37. Cardiac motion is complex, involving translational movements of the whole heart along with the diaphragm during respiration, as well as LV deformation—*shortening, thickening,* and *twisting* during systole.

Deformation Parameters in Myocardial Ischemia II

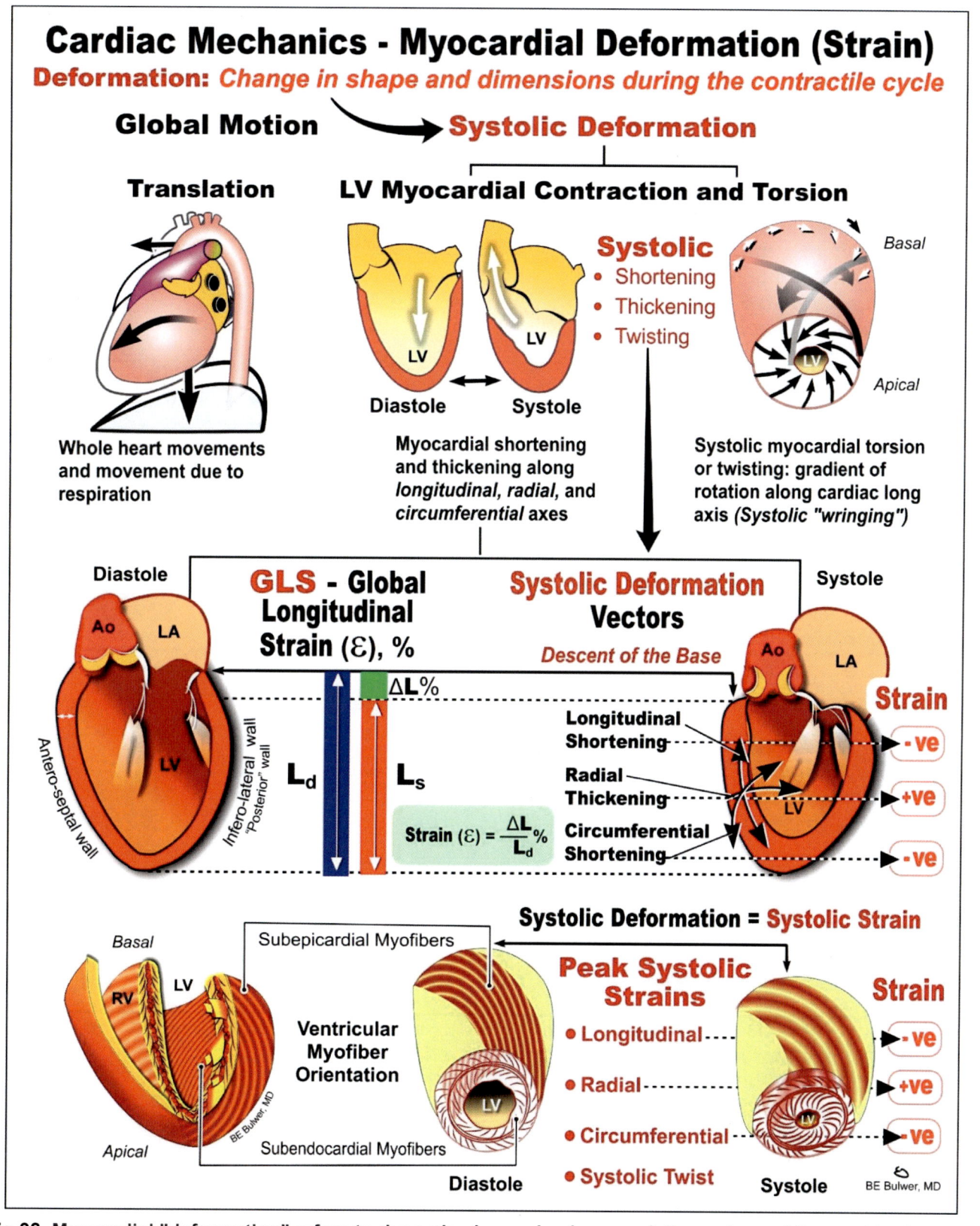

Fig 38. Myocardial "deformation" refers to dynamic change in shape and dimensions of the ventricular walls during the contractile cycle. The extent or magnitude of this change is called **strain**. The rate of this change is called the **strain rate**. *Bottom panel:* Such myocardial deformation that can be measured along four axes using deformation imaging—speckle tracking echocardiography (STE) and tissue Doppler imaging (TDI).

Echo Modality Options in Myocardial Assessment I

Tissue Doppler Imaging and Speckle Tracking Echocardiography Compared

Utility: *For Assessment of Myocardial Systolic and Diastolic Mechanics or Deformation): Velocity, Strain Rate, Displacement, and Strain*

Tissue Doppler Imaging (TDI)

Advantage
- High Temporal Resolution (Higher Frame Rates) compared to STE
- Better Spatial Resolution (image quality) compared to STE
- Wider Availability
- Real-time Analysis

Limitations
- Angle-Dependent (Doppler)
- Manual placement of Sample Volume
- Strain is derived from TDI velocity
- Measures Regional Strain only, not global strain as with STE
- Difficulty assessing Apical LV Segments
- 1-Dimensional Measurements
- Greater Interobserver Variability
- More Sensitive to Signal Noise

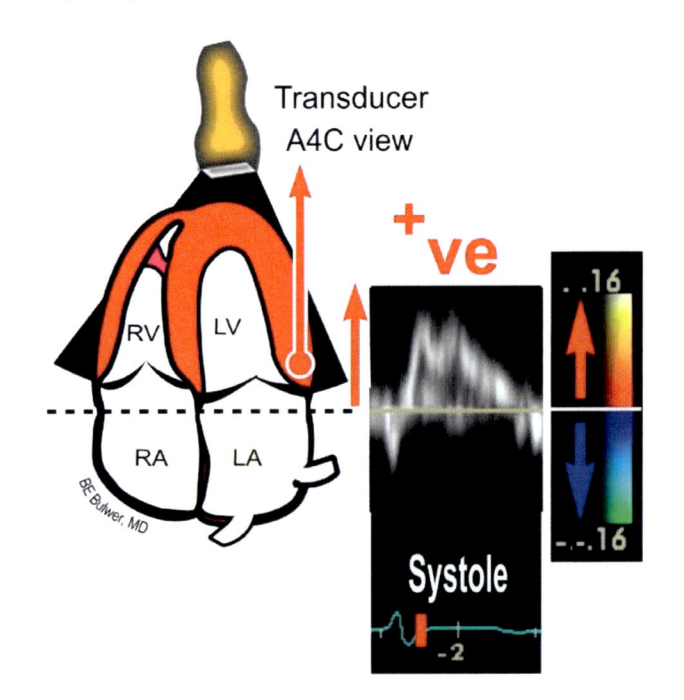

Speckle Tracking Echocardiography (STE)

Advantage
- Angle-Independent
- Measures Deformation (Strain and Strain Rate) in 3-Dimensions: 2D STE and 3D STE
- 3D STE more accurate than 2D STE
- Measures Both Regional and Global Strain
- Semi-Automated Processing
- Less affected by Artifacts
- Less interobserver variability
- Less Sensitive to Signal Noise

Limitations
- Speckle Quality Dependent: Better Image Quality Needed i.e. Spatial Resolution - both Axial and Lateral
- Speckle Tracking affected by Cardiac Motion
- Lower Temporal Resolution (Lower Frame Rates) compared to TDI
- Lower Spatial Resolution (compared to TDI)
- Must Ensure Tracking for Each Myocardial Segment

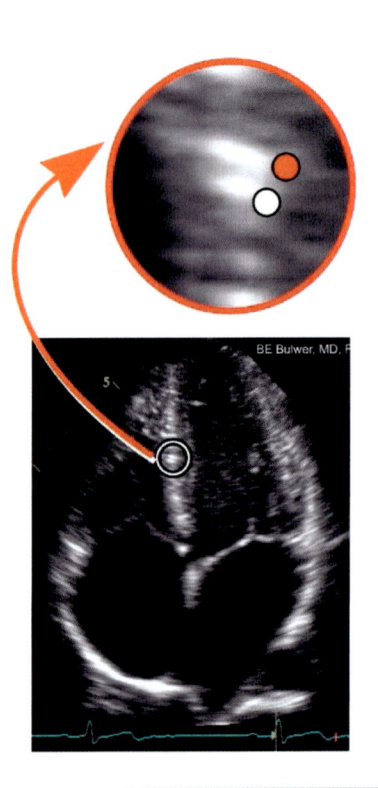

Fig 39. Tissue Doppler Imaging (TDI) and speckle tracking echocardiography (STE) are sensitive measures of myocardial function. They have established utility in the assessment of systolic and diastolic function in patients with coronary artery disease. Compare with Figs. 40-54.

Echo Modality Options in Myocardial Assessment II

Speckle Tracking Echocardiography (STE) Protocol: Global Longitudinal Strain (GLS)

Optimal Image Acquision
- High quality images (>40 frames/sec): Apical views:
- A3C (ALAX), A4C, A2C
- Identification of LV apex, endocardial border, regions
- of interest
- Evaluate tracking quality

Mark Aortic Valve Closure (AVC)
- Select CW Doppler of Aortic Valve
- Identify AVC click
- Choose event timing
- Place pointer on AVC closure click

Launch STE Software
- Start with the A3C (ALAX) view, then A4C, A2C
  Start with the A3C-ALAX View
- Select the best A3C beat of 3-beat loop
- Trim down to a 1-cycle loop
- Select and label as A3C/ALAX
  Select Region of Interest for Tracking
  For global longitudinal strain (GLS) of LV:
- For annular points: position at junction of mitral annulus and LV wall
- For apical points: subendocardium of apical segments

Analyze STE - Ensure Accurate Tracking
- Begn with analysis of the A3C (ALAX) view
  Start with the A3C-ALAX View
- Ensure accurate tracking
- Analyze and accept GLS values
  Repeat above for A4C and A2C Views

Final GLS Report
- Generate report following analysis of above views
- Record and report GLS: vendor parametric display options

Global Longitudinal Strain Images: *Vendor Variations*

BE Bulwer, MD, FASE

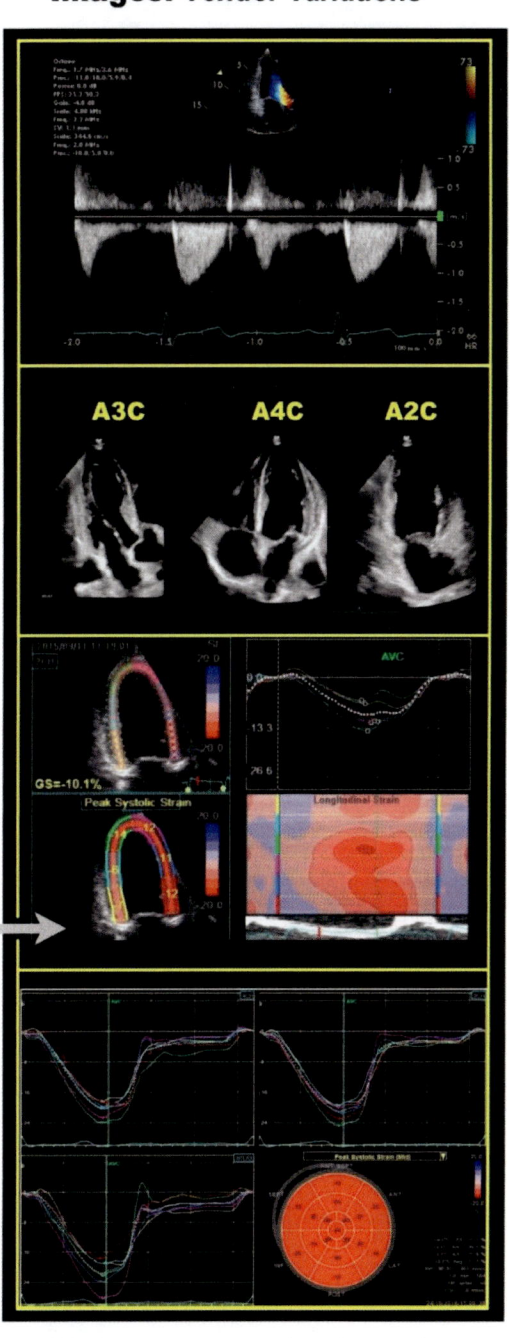

Fig 40. Speckle tracking echocardiography (STE) has gained popularity in the assessment of myocardial function in patients with coronary artery disease. It has significant advantages over TDI assessment of myocardial function. Chief among them are its angle-independence and post-processing software algorithms for assessment of all myocardial segments. See Figs. 42, 47-54.

Global Longitudinal LV Strain and Strain Rate I

Longitudinal Systolic Strain
- Global Longitudinal Shortening -

Strain Rate (SR) s^{-1} **Strain (ε), %**

A4C — RV, LV — L_d — Diastole — L_s — Systole — L_d — L_s — ΔL %

Longitudinal Systolic Strain (ε)

$$\varepsilon_{\text{Strain}} = \frac{L_{\text{systole}} - L_{\text{diastole}}}{L_{\text{diastole}}} = \frac{\Delta L}{L_d} \%$$

Systolic Strain: (-) Negative values   Normal range: -15-25% (SD 5% - 7%)

BE Bulwer, MD, FASE

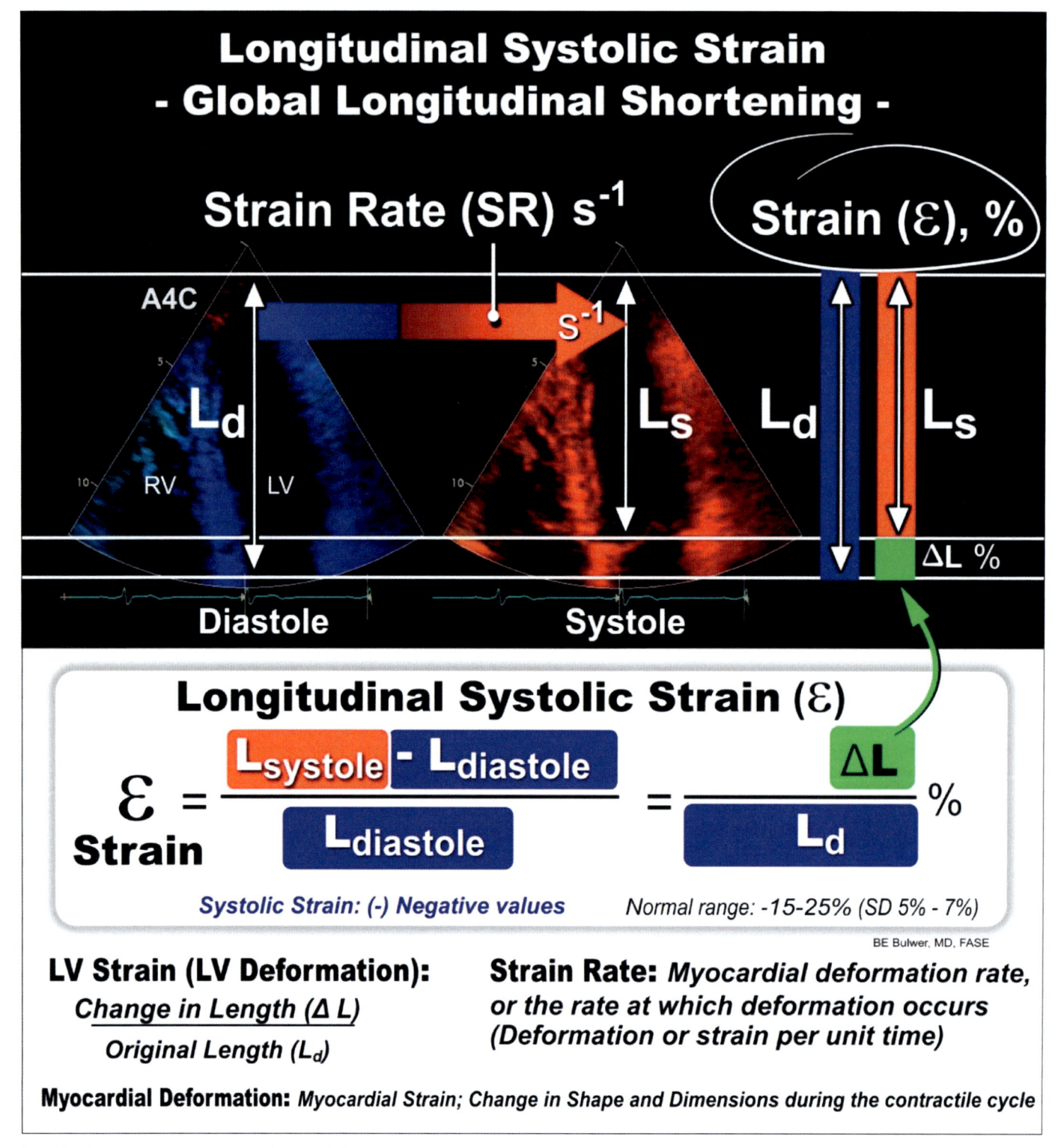

LV Strain (LV Deformation):
$$\frac{\text{Change in Length } (\Delta L)}{\text{Original Length } (L_d)}$$

Strain Rate: *Myocardial deformation rate, or the rate at which deformation occurs (Deformation or strain per unit time)*

Myocardial Deformation: *Myocardial Strain; Change in Shape and Dimensions during the contractile cycle*

Fig. 41. Tissue Doppler imaging (TDI)-derived longitudinal systolic strain rate (SR) and strain (ε). Longitudinal systolic strain (ε_L) is the total amount of LV shortening that occurs during ventricular systole *(above right)*. It is a comparison of the diastolic length (L_{diastole} or L_d) to the systolic length (L_{systole} or L_s) and as represented in the equation shown. The rate of this change in length, or the spatial velocity gradient, is the **strain rate** (**SR**) *(above left)*. See Figs, 37-40

Global Longitudinal LV Strain and Strain Rate II

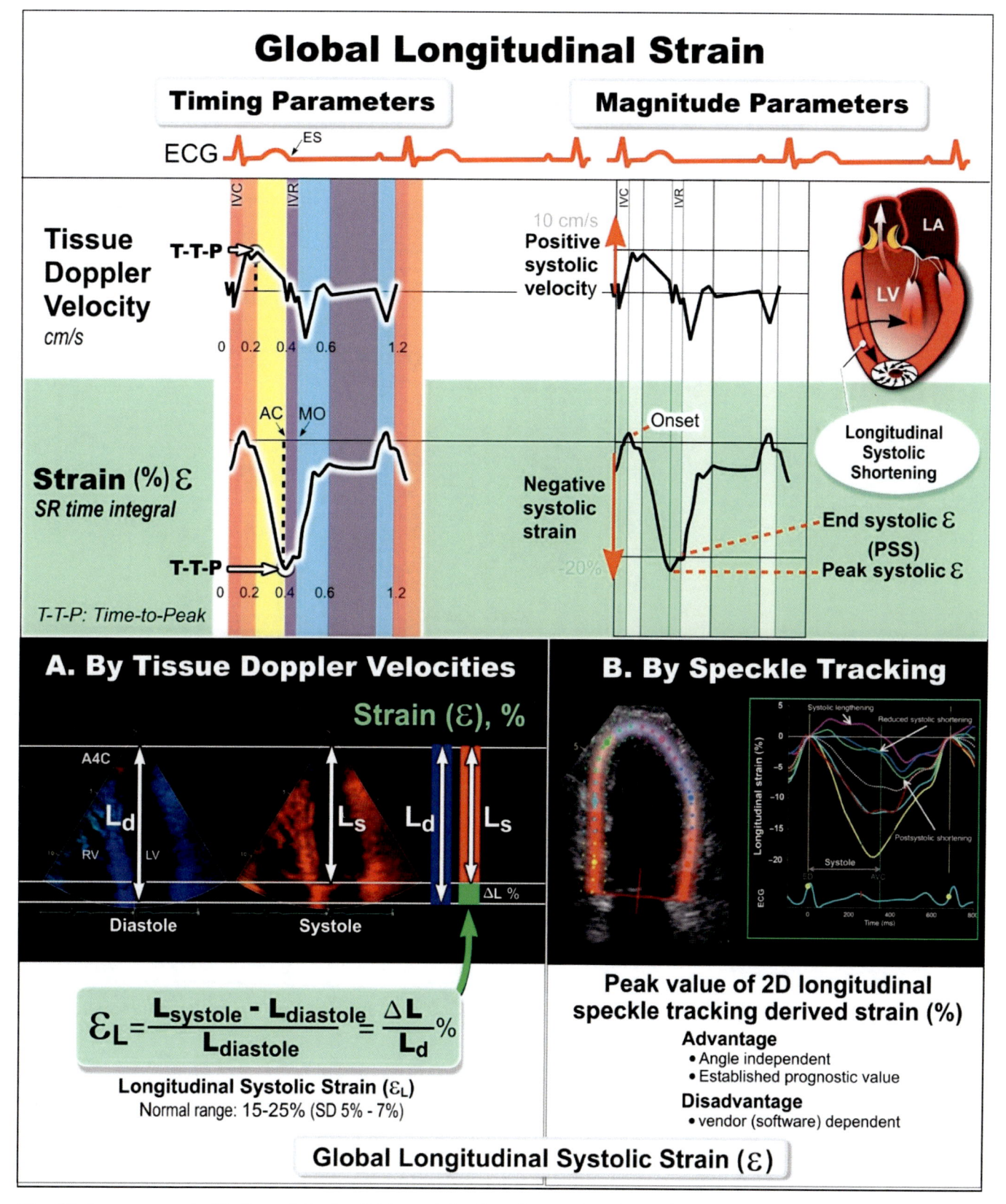

Fig. 42. Assessment of left ventricular (LV) systolic function using tissue Doppler imaging (TDI) and derived global longitudinal strain *(top panel and below left)*. **Speckle tracking imaging** has gained popularity, because unlike tissue Doppler, it is angle-independent and can better assess deformation of the apical LV segments. *See* Figs, 39, 40, 47-54.

TDI-derived Global Longitudinal Strain Rate I

Tissue Doppler Imaging (TDI) and Longitudinal Strain Rate

Longitudinal Velocity Gradients by TDI

Tissue Doppler (TDI): Septal wall of the LV

Tissue Doppler (TDI): Antero-lateral wall of the LV

Velocity gradient from Base to Apex

S^1 E^1 A^1

A4C view

Longitudinal TDI-derived Strain Rate (SR)

$$SR = \frac{V_2 - V_1}{d} \; (s^{-1})$$

Normal range: 1.0/s - 1.4/s; (SD 0.5/s - 0.6/s)

Spatial Velocity Gradient (Δv)

IVC AVO AVC MVO E MVC

- Strain Rate (SR) is the Velocity Difference ($V_2 - V_1$) per unit of Distance (d) (or Length) between two points in the myocardium (ventricular wall), i.e., a *Spatial Velocity Gradient*

- Longitudinal SR measures the *Spatial Velocity Gradient* from base to apex in the longitudinal axis.

BE Bulwer, MD, FASE

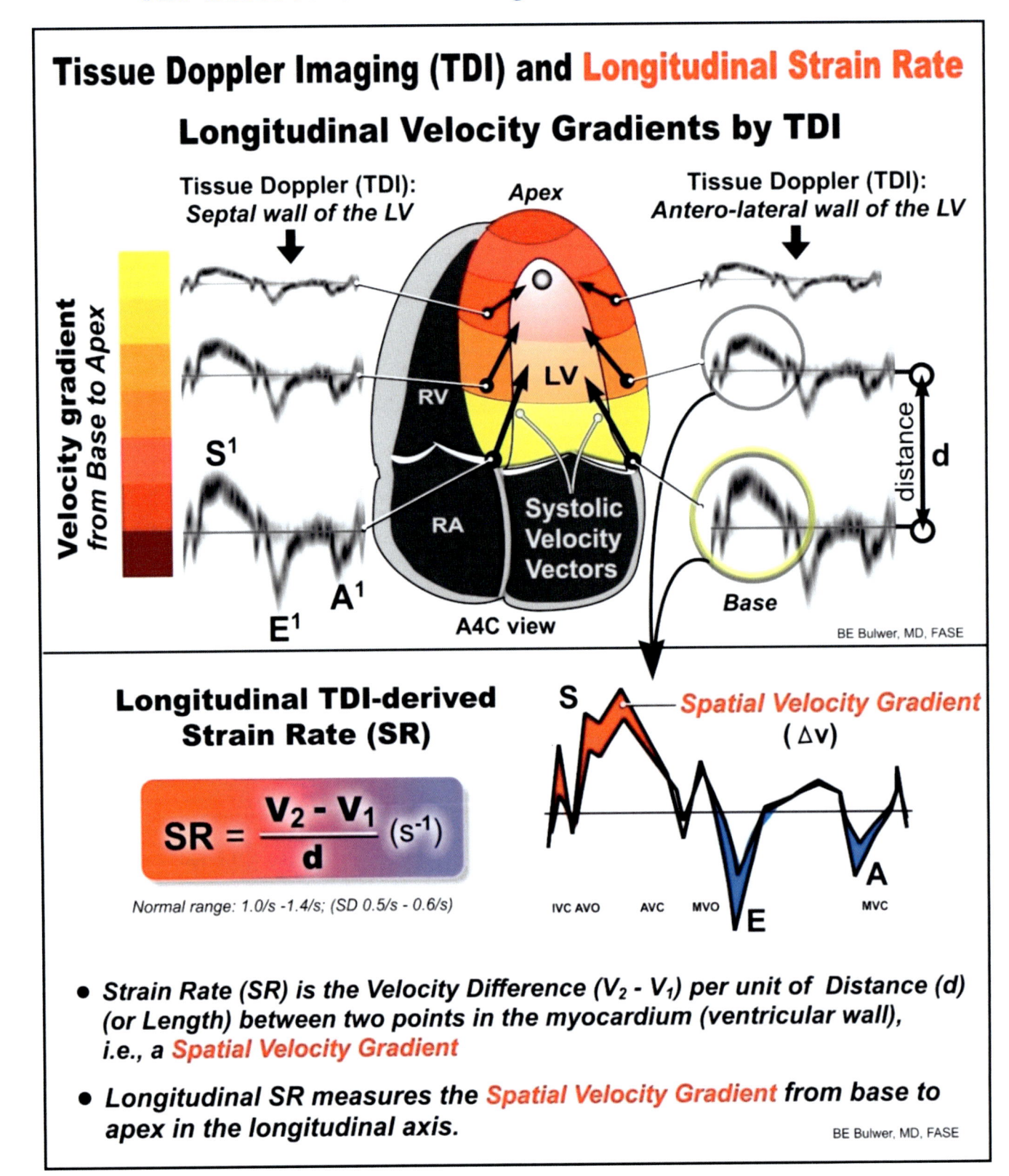

Fig. 43. Tissue Doppler imaging (TDI) of the left ventricular (LV) myocardium showing a velocity differential or gradient from LV apex to base. Note the highest myocardial velocities at the base, which progressively diminish toward the relatively stationary apex. Note also the corresponding color-coded myocardial velocities *(upper panel)*. The difference between TDI velocities at two points, separated by distance (d) within the LV myocardium during ventricular systolic shortening can be quantified. Compare with Figs. 37-48.

# TDI-derived Global Longitudinal Strain Rate II

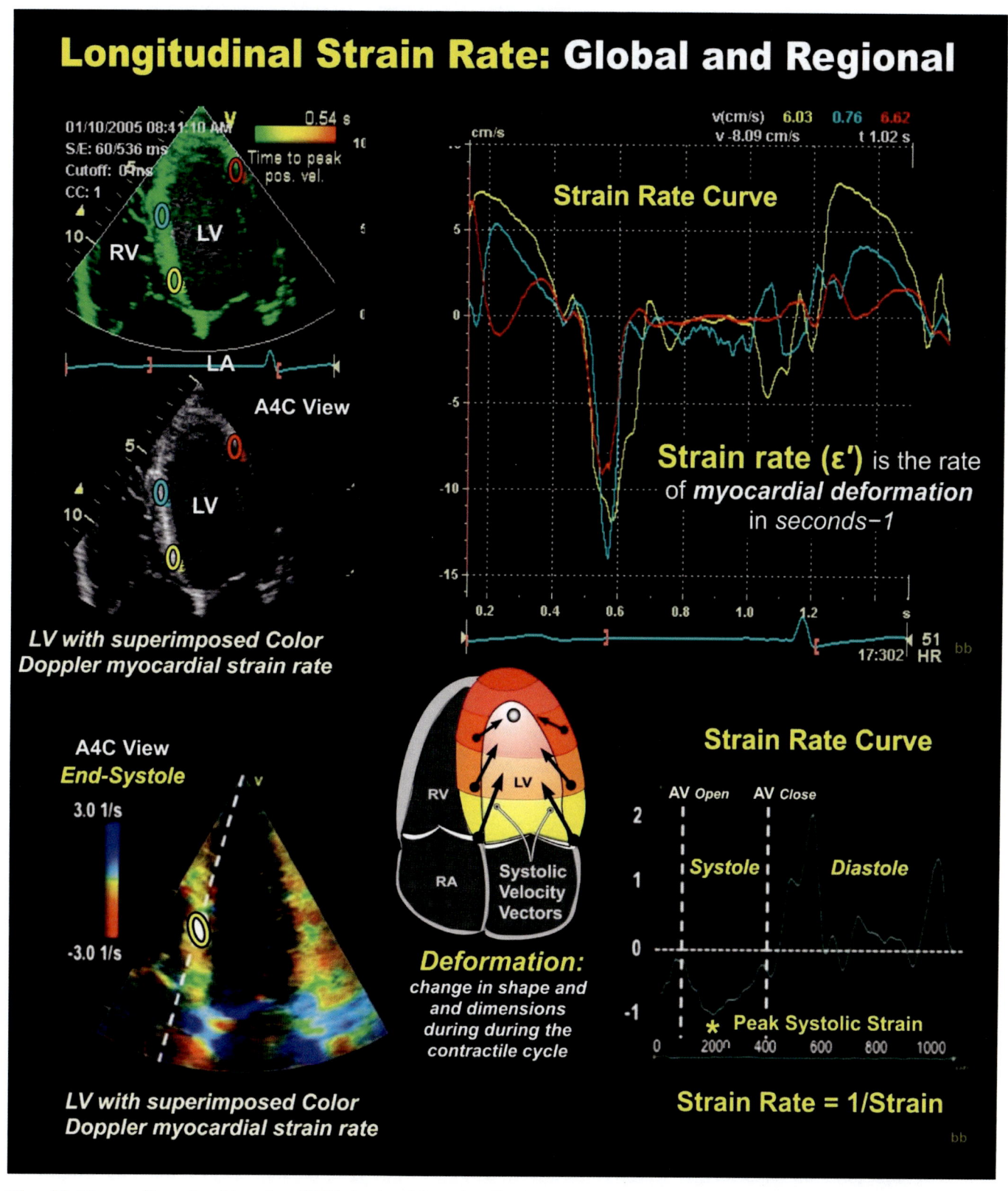

Fig. 44. Tissue Doppler imaging (TDI) derived longitudinal strain rate (SR) measured on the apical four-chamber (A4C) view. The longitudinal SR is derived from the difference in myocardial velocities measured at two different points within the LV myocardium. Longitudinal strain represents the integration of SR with over time. Compare with Figs. 37-48.

TDI-derived Measures of Systolic Function I

Longitudinal Systolic TDI-derived Measures

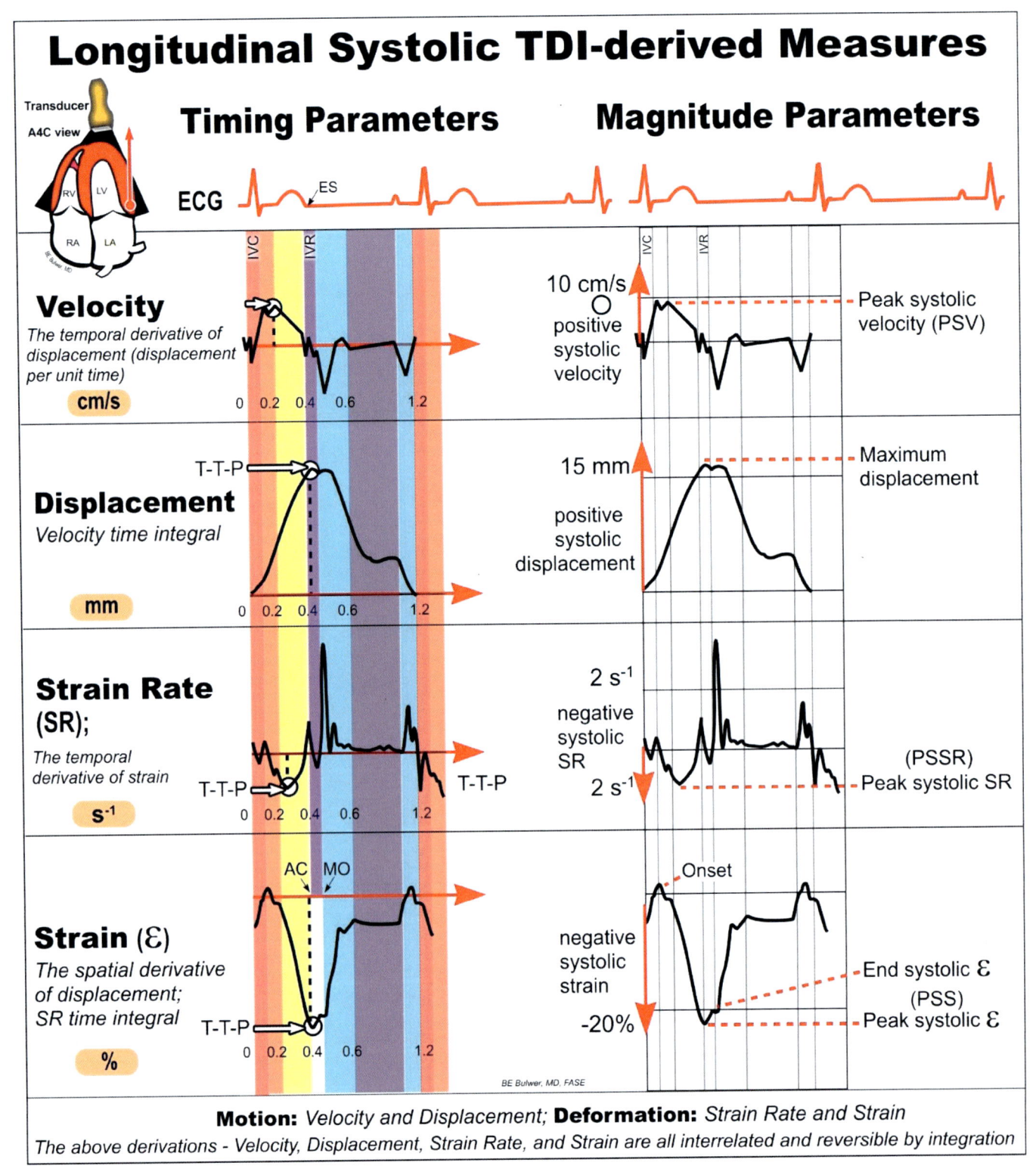

Timing Parameters | **Magnitude Parameters**

Transducer A4C view

ECG — ES

Velocity — The temporal derivative of displacement (displacement per unit time) — cm/s
- 10 cm/s positive systolic velocity
- Peak systolic velocity (PSV)

Displacement — Velocity time integral — mm
- T-T-P
- 15 mm positive systolic displacement
- Maximum displacement

Strain Rate (SR) — The temporal derivative of strain — s⁻¹
- T-T-P
- 2 s⁻¹ negative systolic SR
- 2 s⁻¹ (PSSR) Peak systolic SR

Strain (ε) — The spatial derivative of displacement; SR time integral — %
- AC MO
- T-T-P
- negative systolic strain
- −20%
- Onset
- End systolic ε (PSS)
- Peak systolic ε

Motion: Velocity and Displacement; **Deformation:** Strain Rate and Strain
The above derivations - Velocity, Displacement, Strain Rate, and Strain are all interrelated and reversible by integration

Fig 45. **Tissue Doppler imaging (TDI)-derived parameters**, starting from top to bottom: **1) Velocity, 2) Displacement** (velocity × time), **3) Strain rate (SR)** rate of myocardial deformation, and **4) Strain (ε)**—change in length-shortening or thickening. Tissue Doppler velocities (by TDI) assess myocardial motion, but does not distinguish motion of healthy versus nonviable myocardium that moves passively. **Strain (ε) and strain rate (SR) measures** *can distinguish true contractile tissue motion from motion simply due to tethering.* These measures have clinical utility in patients with coronary artery disease. **AC**—aortic valve closure; **ES**—end systole; **IVC**—isovolumetric contraction; **IVR**—isovolumetric relaxation; **MO**—mitral valve opening; **S**—peak systolic velocity.

Myocardial Longitudinal Strain and Strain Rate I

Myocardial Deformation: Strain Rate and Strain

Myocardial "deformation" refers to dynamic changes in shape and dimensions of the myocardium (ventricular walls) during the contractile cycle. The extent or magnitude of this change is called STRAIN. The rate of this change is called the STRAIN RATE.

Strain Rate (SR) s^{-1}

The temporal derivative of strain

- Strain Rate shows multiple rapid shifts in direction of deformation
- These rapid shifts make Strain Rate better suited for timing events.

Strain (ε) %

Spatial derivative of displacement; SR time integral

- Note the corresponding peaks and troughs of both the Strain Rate and Strain Rate curves
- Strain remains negative throughout the cardiac cycle

AVC: aortic valve closure; AVO: aortic valve opening; IVC: isovolumetric contraction; IVR: isovolumetric relaxation; MVC: mitral valve closure; MVO: mitral valve opening

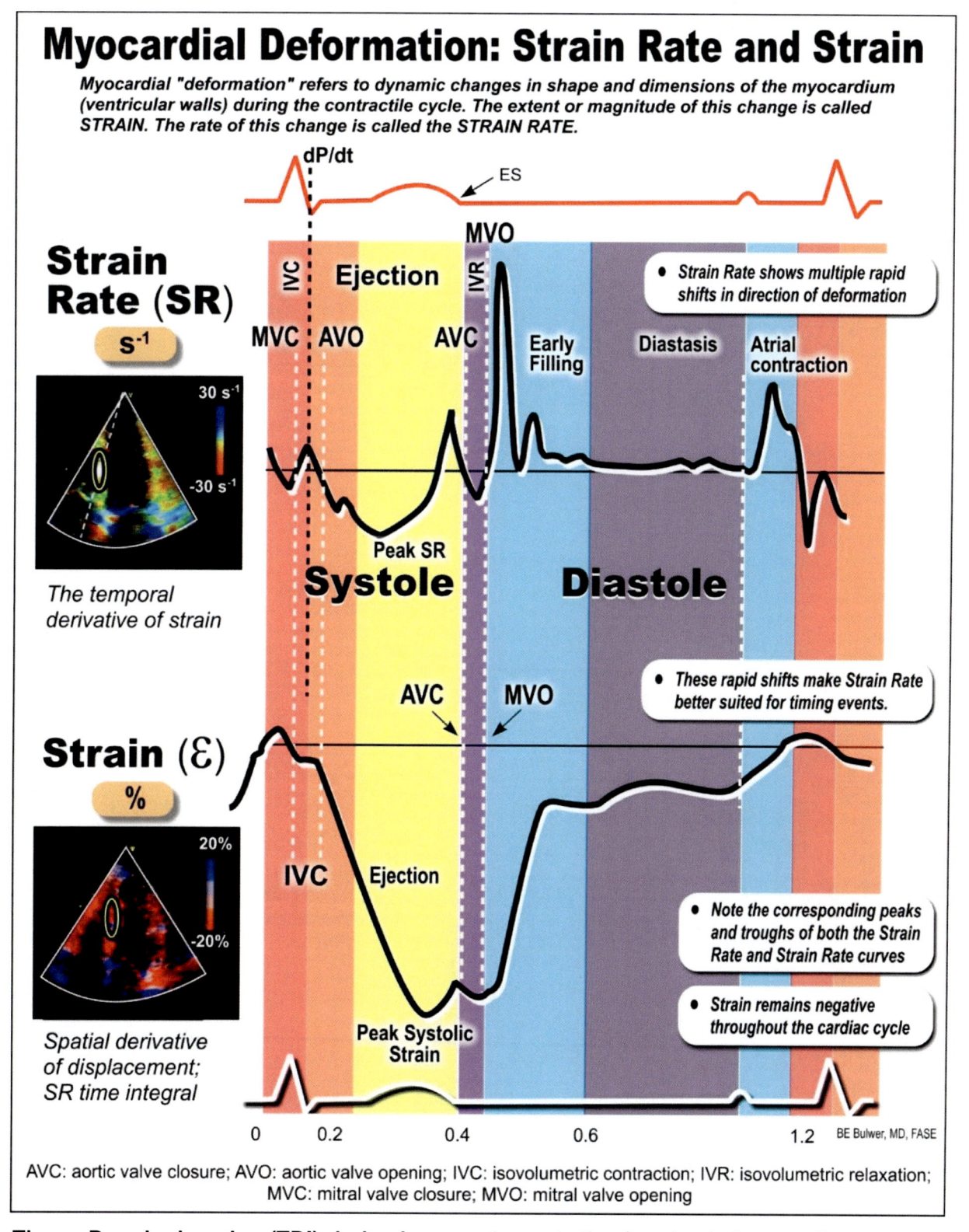

Fig 46. Tissue Doppler imaging (TDI)-derived parameters, starting from top to bottom: **1)** This spatial velocity gradient is the **strain rate (SR)** *(bottom panel)*. The SR curve reflects the rate of longitudinal systolic shortening. **By convention, SR is negative during systole (LV longitudinal shortening) and positive during diastolic (LV longitudinal lengthening)**. The total amount of LV systolic shortening or diastolic lengthening is called **LV longitudinal strain (ε)** and is obtained by the integrating the strain rate (SR) curve. Compare with Figs. 37-48.

Myocardial Longitudinal Strain and Strain Rate II

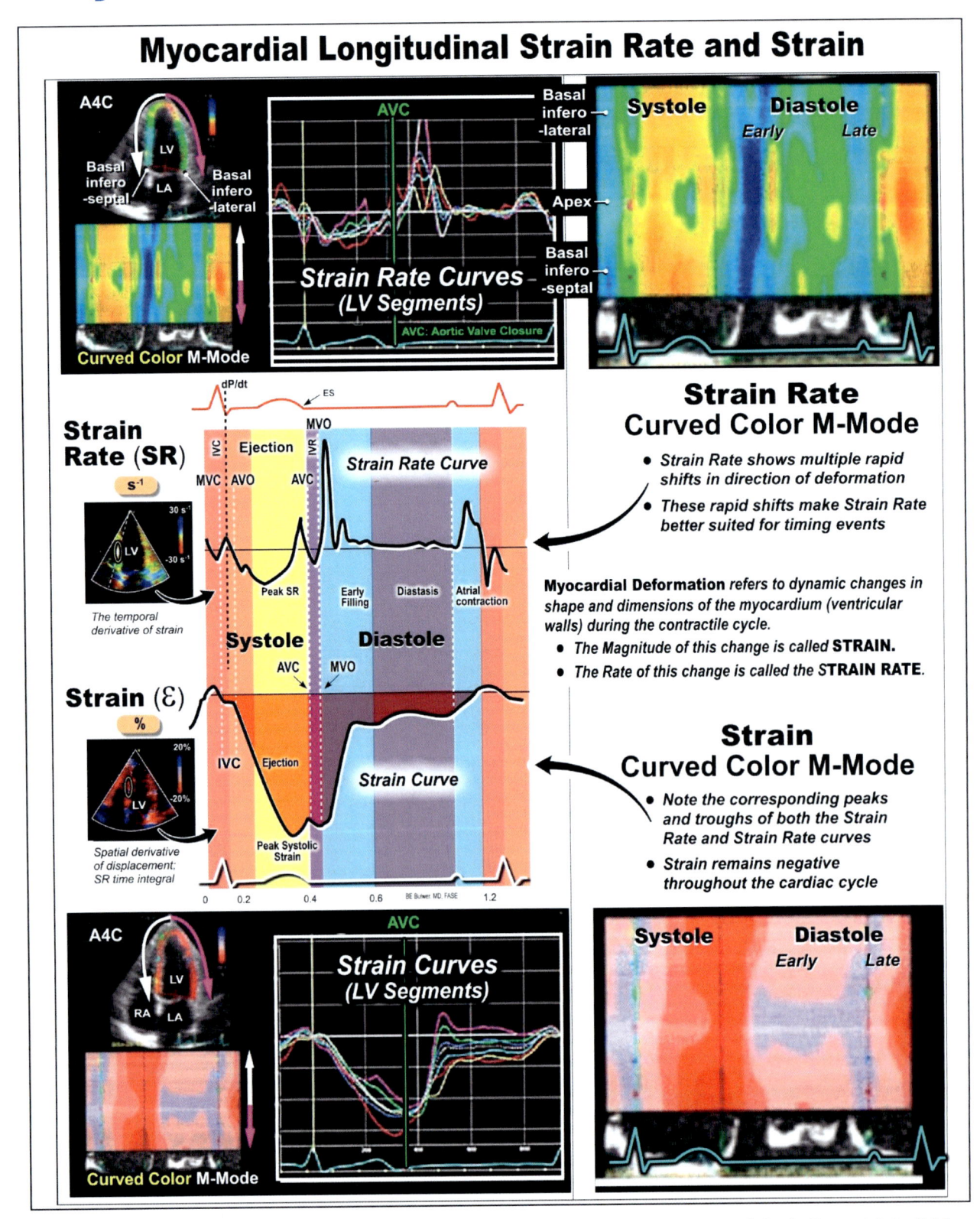

Fig 47. Display options showing longitudinal strain rate *(above)* and strain *(below)* of the left ventricle (LV) on the apical four-chamber (A4C) view. These parameters are useful in patients with suspected or established coronary heart disease. Ischemic myocardium exhibits reduced strain and strain rates. Display options include strain and strain rate curves, as well as curved anatomical color M-mode displays as shown. Compare with Figs. 40, 48-60.

Strain and Strain Rate: Longitudinal, Radial, Circumferential

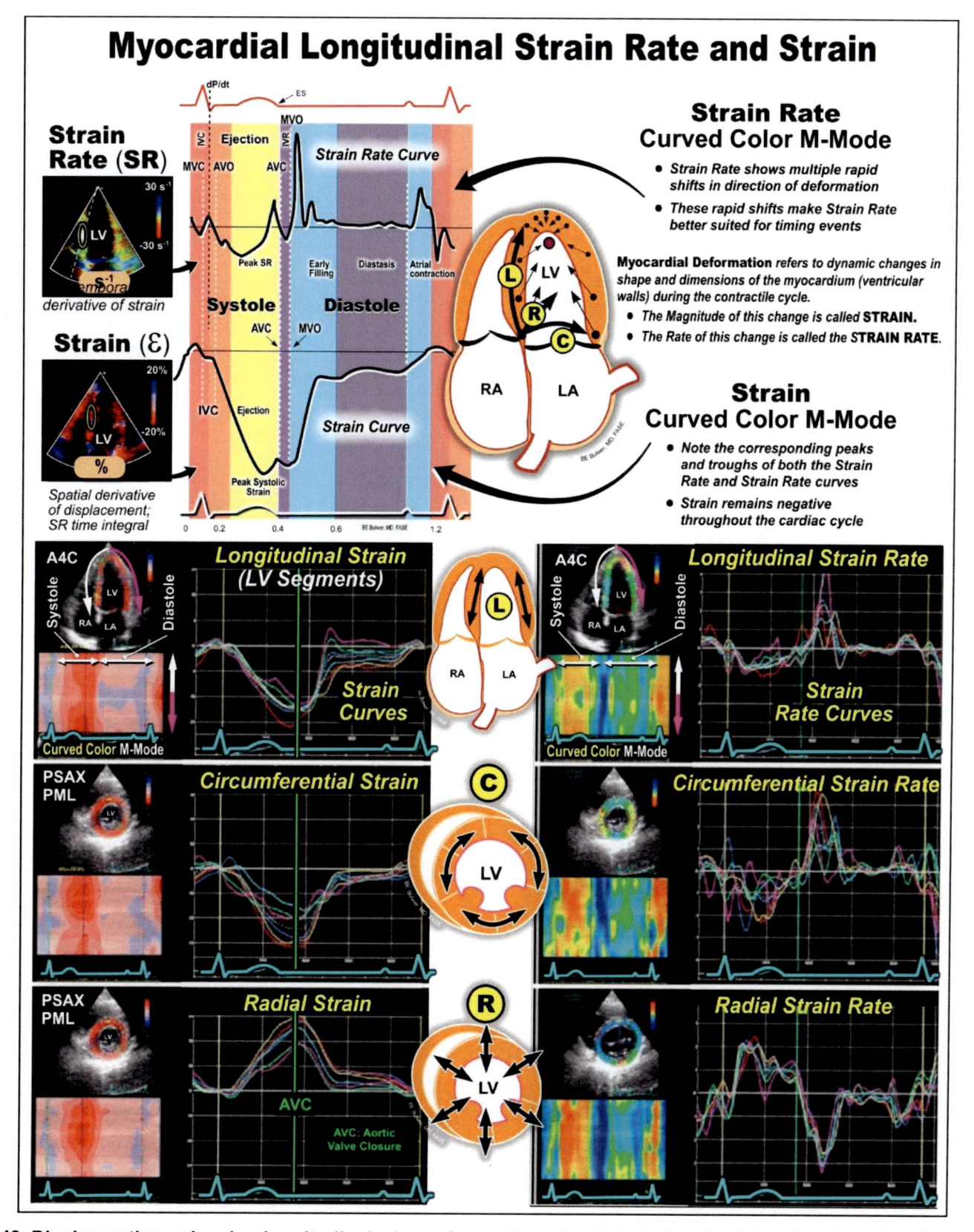

Fig 48. Display options showing longitudinal, circumferential, and radial strain rates *(above)* **and strains** *(below)* **of the left ventricle (LV) on the apical four-chamber (A4C) and short-axis views.** Display options include strain and strain rate curves, as well as curved anatomical color M-mode displays as shown. Compare with Figs. 40, 47-60.

Myocardial Velocities and Display Options I

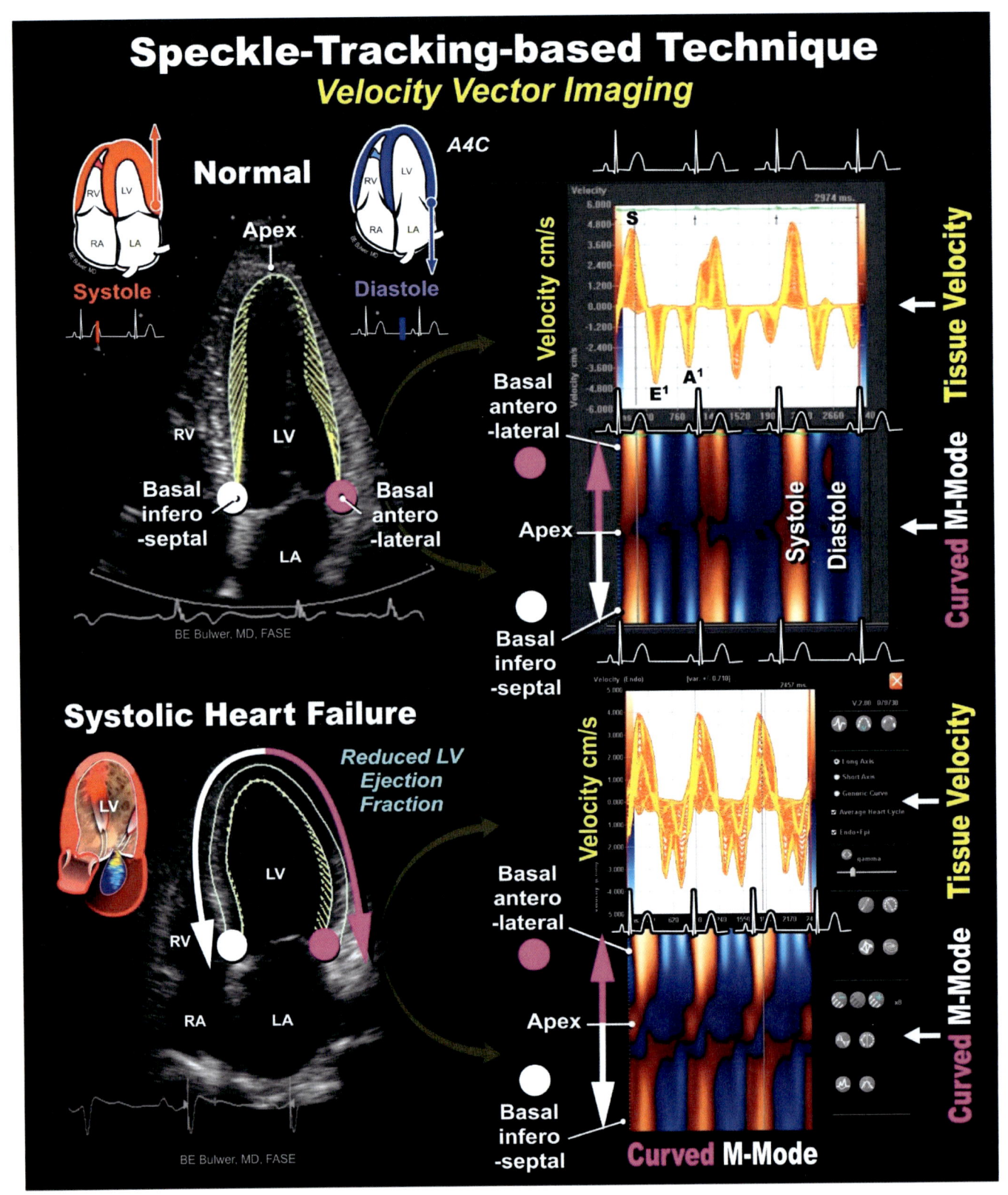

Fig. 49. Speckle tracking imaging (STE)-based technique—Velocity vector imaging (VVI) for assessment and display of myocardial tissue velocities and corresponding curved anatomical color M-mode displays. Compare the parameters in the normal heart *(above)* compared to that with systolic heart failure *(below)*. Compare with Figs. 37-54.

STE-based Myocardial Velocities and Display Options II

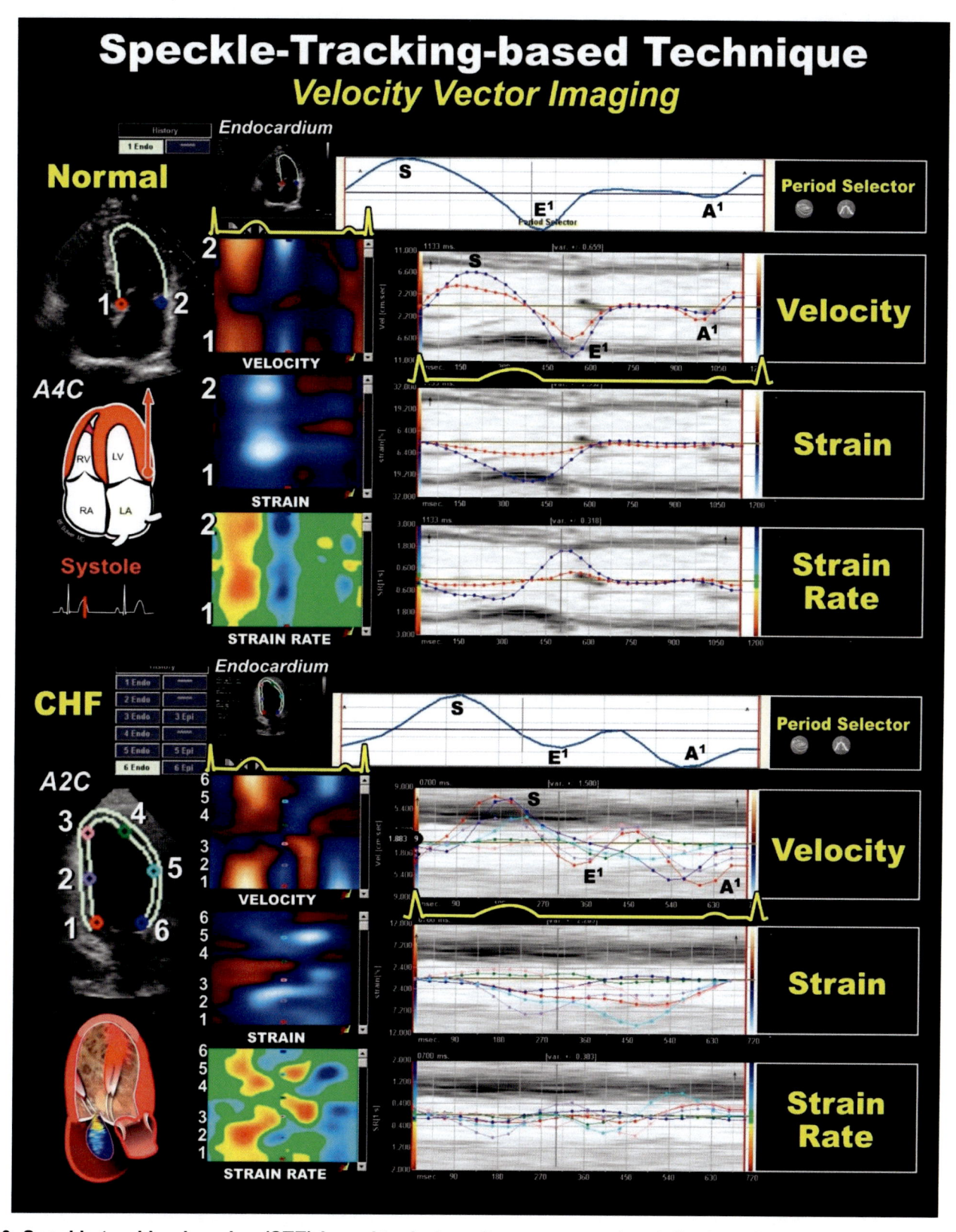

Fig. 50. Speckle tracking imaging (STE)-based technique for assessment and display of myocardial tissue velocities, with derived strain and strain rate. Compare the parameters in the normal heart (above) compared to that with congestive heart failure (CHF) (below). Compare with Figs. 37-54.

Longitudinal, Radial, and Circumferential Strain I

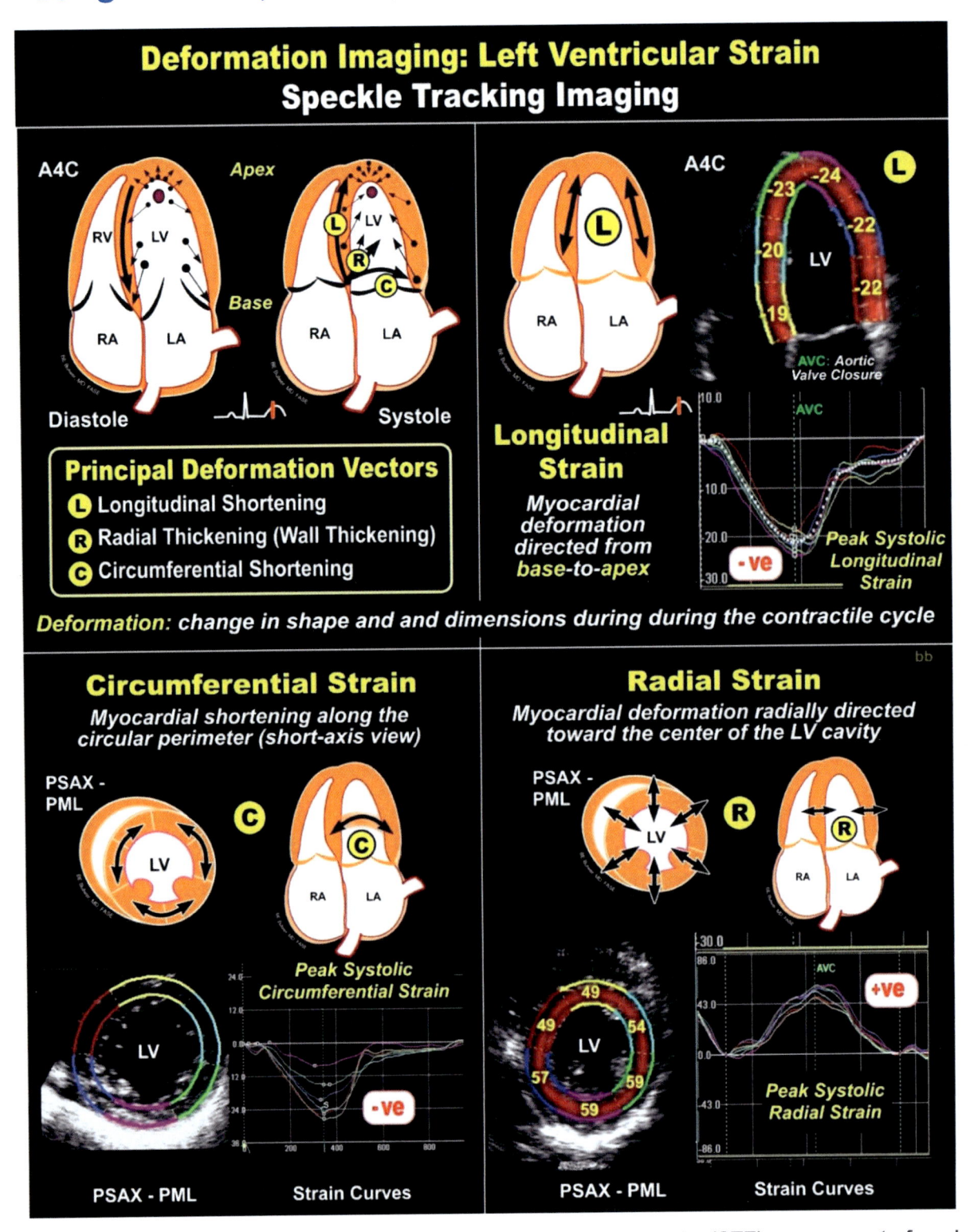

Fig. 51. Myocardial strain imaging using speckle tracking echocardiography (STE) assessment of peak systolic strains along three principal axes of deformation: longitudinal shortening, radial thickening, and circumferential shortening *(above left)*. Global longitudinal strain (GLS) *(above right)*, global circumferential strain (GCS) *(below left)*, and global radial strain (GRS) *(below right)*.

Note (i) the **direction of the vectors (arrows)** along which the different strain parameters measured, (ii) the **segmental strain values** (except for circumferential strain) superimposed on the LV myocardial images, and (iii) the **regional strain curves and peak systolic strain**. Compare with Figs. 37-40, 47-60.

Longitudinal, Radial, and Circumferential Strain II

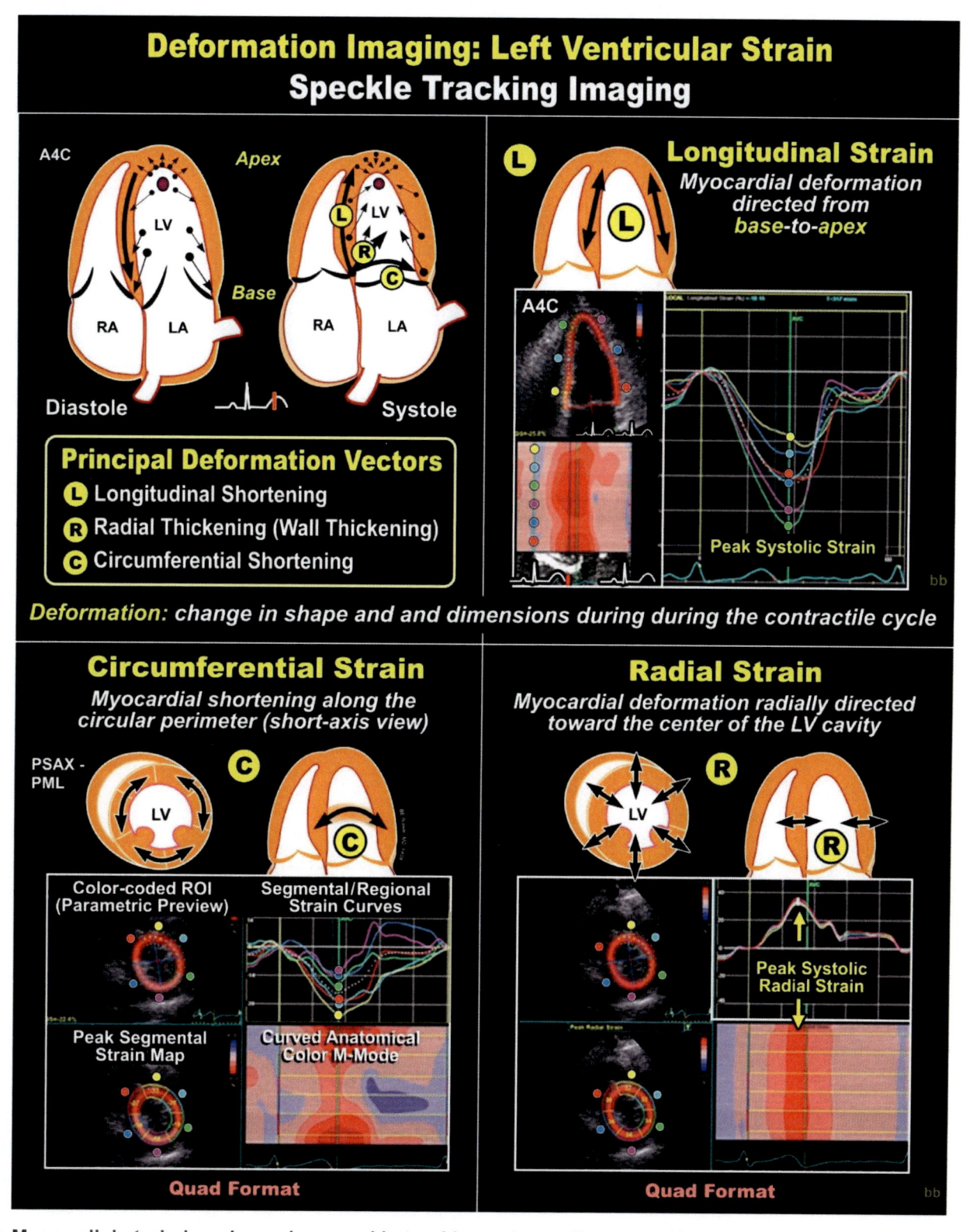

Fig. 52. Myocardial strain imaging using speckle tracking echocardiography (STE) assessment of peak systolic strains along three principal axes of deformation as in previous figure. The "quad format" is a popular proprietary display that uses four complementary parametric displays: (i) color-coded region of interest, (ii) segmental or regional strain curves, (iii) peak segmental strain, and (iv) curved anatomical color M-mode display format. **Compare with Figs. 37-40, 47-60.**

Circumferential Strain and Strain Rate I

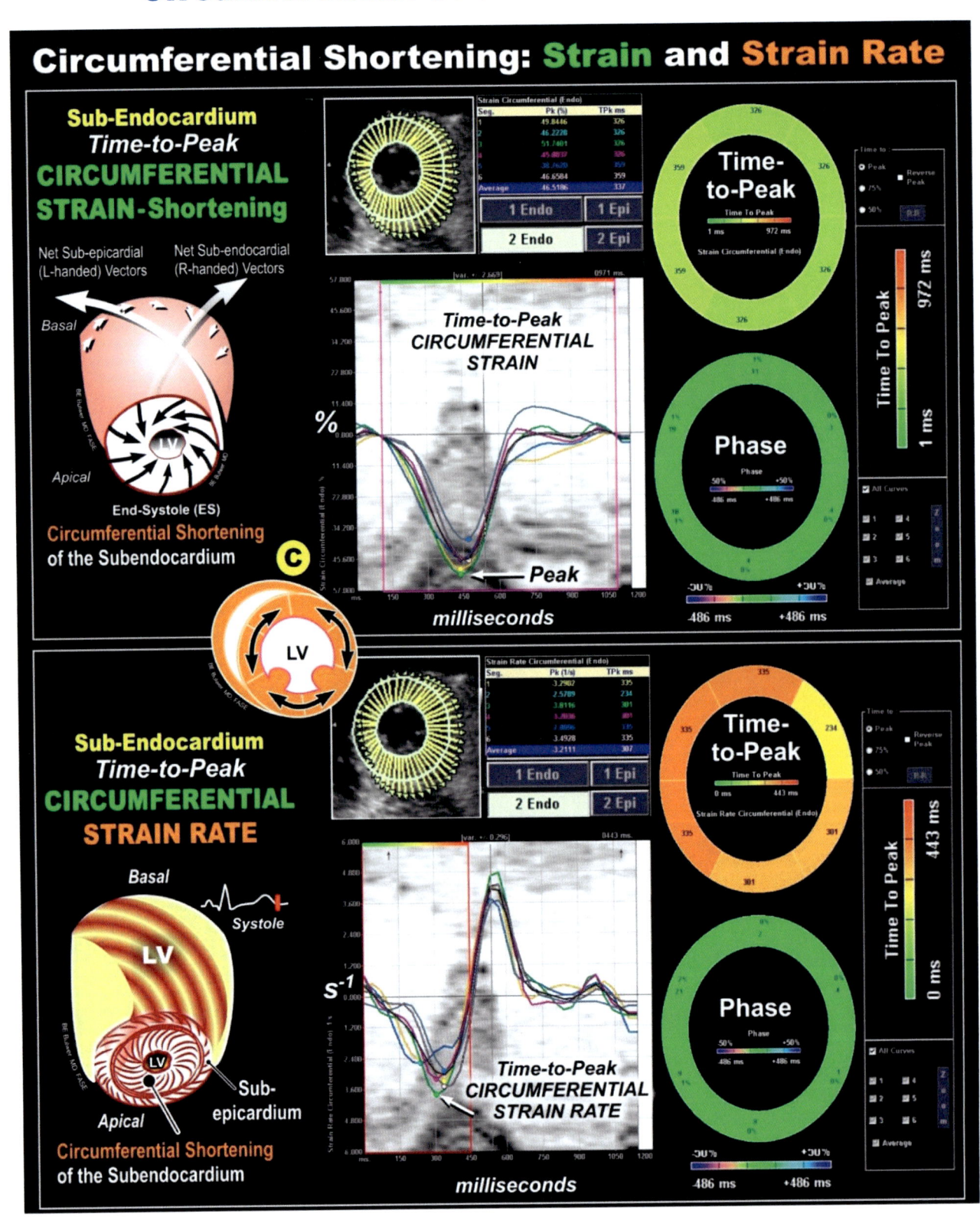

Fig. 53. Circumferential shortening of the left ventricle (LV) by speckle tracking echocardiography (STE). Deformation of the LV along the circumferential axis can be assessed by circumferential strain and strain rate parameters as shown. These can be displayed as strain and strain rate curves *(center)* with complementary color-coded parametric displays showing time-to-peak circumferential strain and strain rate *(right)*.

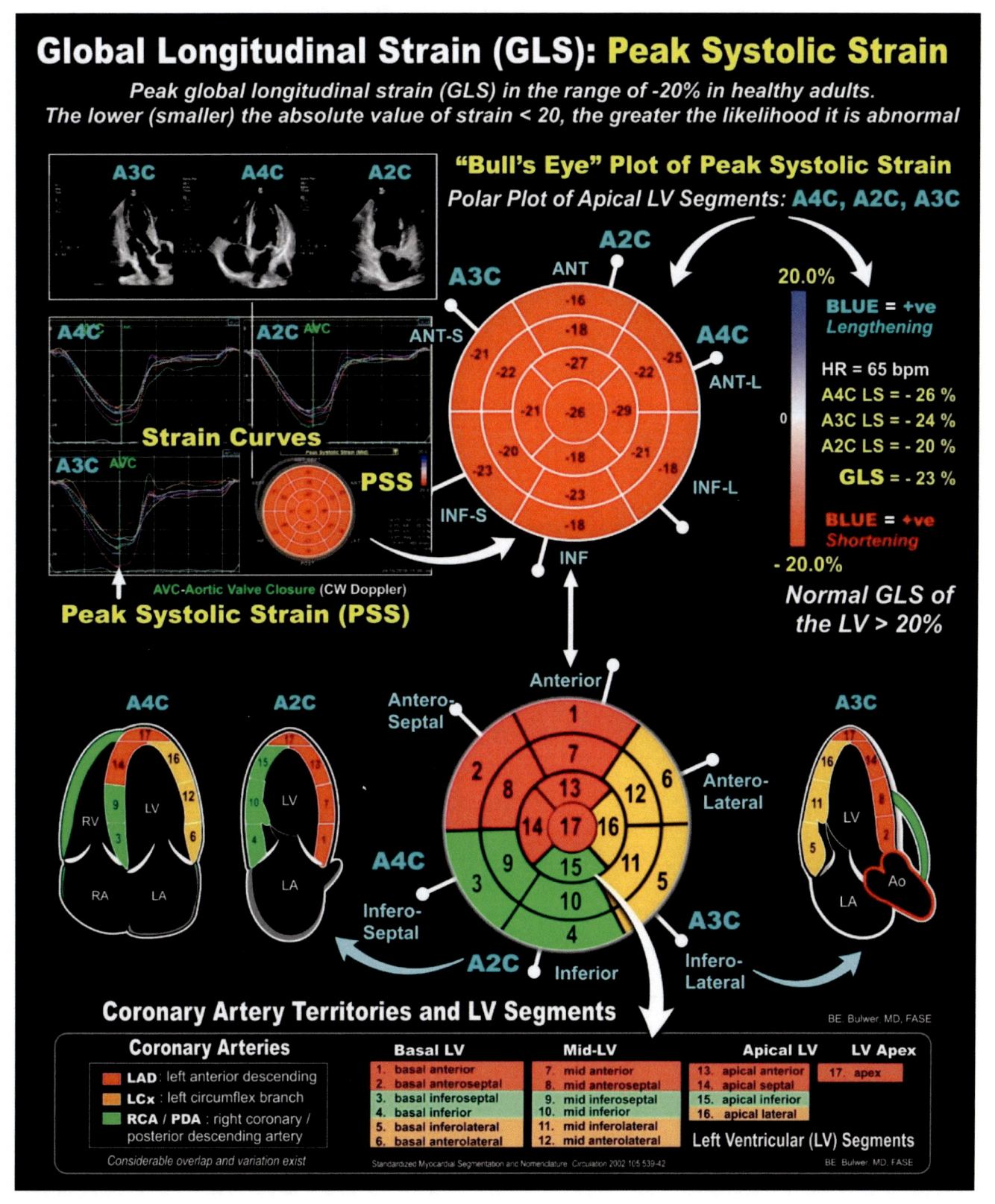

Figure 54. Global longitudinal strain (GLS) displayed using a bull's eye plot of peak systolic strain (PSS) on the 17-segment model of the LV walls. Speckle tracking echocardiography (STE) of the three apical views (upper left) is displayed both as segmental strain curves (upper left) or using the bull's eye format. Compare with Figs. 5-8, 38-40, 55-59.

LV Strain Imaging: Clinical Applications

Utility of Strain (Deformation) Imaging in LV Function Assessment

Clinical Applications

- Coronary Artery Disease
- LV Dysfunction; Heart Failure
- LV Hypertrophy; Cardiomyopathy
- Cancer Therapy Related Dysfunction
- Valvular Heart Disease

Global Function: Global Longitudinal Strain (GLS) *(Absolute values)*

Very Severe	Severe	Reduced	Borderline	Normal	Supra-Normal
GLS < 8%	GLS < 12%	GLS < 12-16%	GLS 16-18%	GLS 18-20%	GLS >18-20%

Reference: JACC Cardiovasc Imaging. 2018;11(2 Pt 1):260-274.

Regional Function - Pattern Recognition

Bull's Eye PolarPlot: LV Segments, Coronary Artery Territories

- **LAD**: left anterior descending
- **LCx**: left circumflex branch
- **RCA / PDA**: right coronary / posterior descending artery

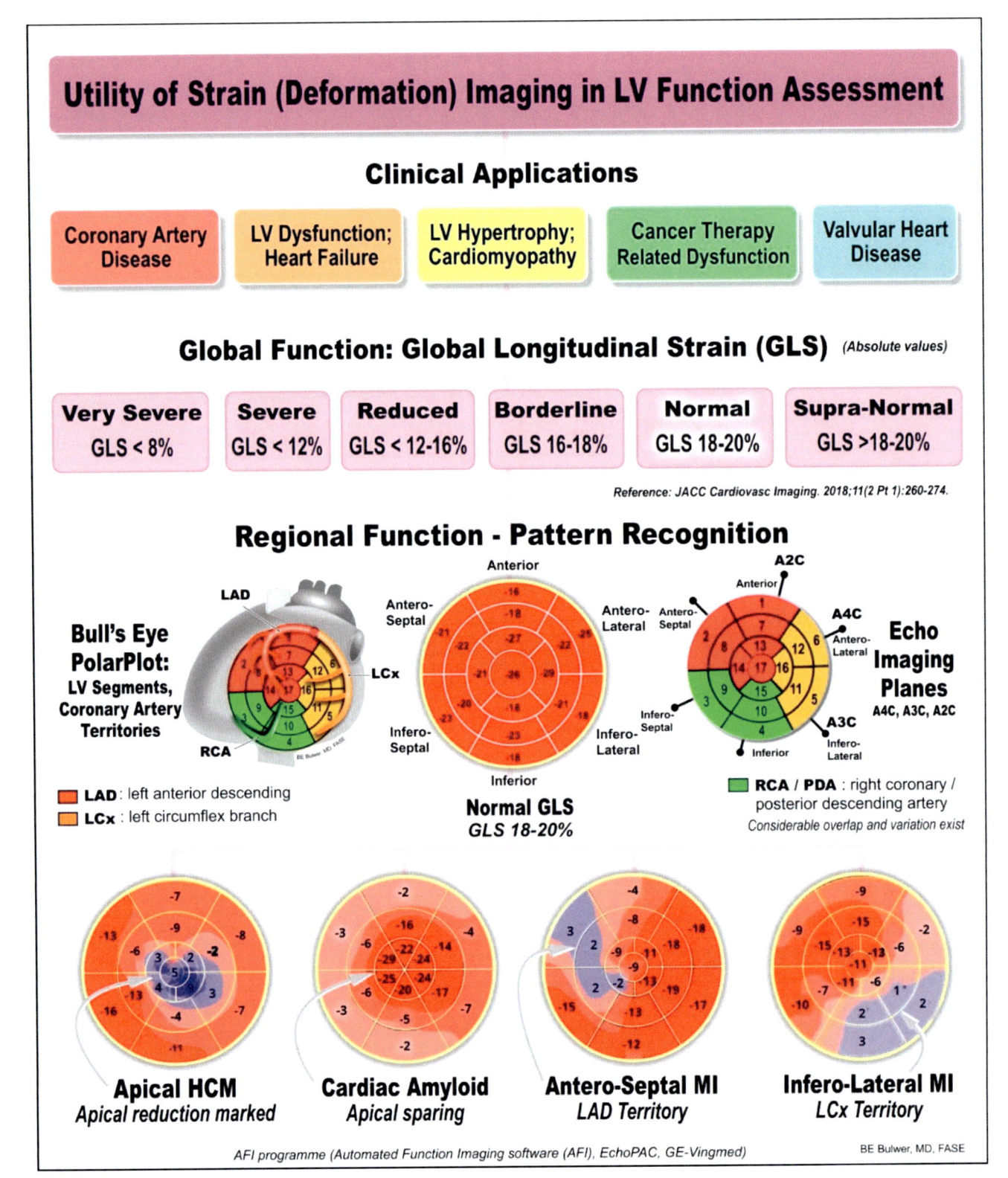

Considerable overlap and variation exist

Normal GLS — GLS 18-20%

Echo Imaging Planes — A4C, A3C, A2C

- **Apical HCM** — Apical reduction marked
- **Cardiac Amyloid** — Apical sparing
- **Antero-Septal MI** — LAD Territory
- **Infero-Lateral MI** — LCx Territory

AFI programme (Automated Function Imaging software (AFI), EchoPAC, GE-Vingmed)

BE Bulwer, MD, FASE

Fig. 55. Clinical applications and display of global longitudinal strain (GLS) displayed using a bull's eye format representing the left ventricular (LV) segments. This display format is excellent for the assessment of regional ventricular function and pattern recognition in ischemia and non-ischemic heart disease. Compare with Figs. 5-8, 38-40, 55-59.

Coronary Artery Territories and Ischemic Patterns I

Wall Motion Assessment: LAD Territory

17-Segment Model of LV (ASE-AHA)

Considerable overlap and variation exist

- **LAD**: left anterior descending
- **LCx**: left circumflex branch
- **RCA / PDA**: right coronary / posterior descending artery

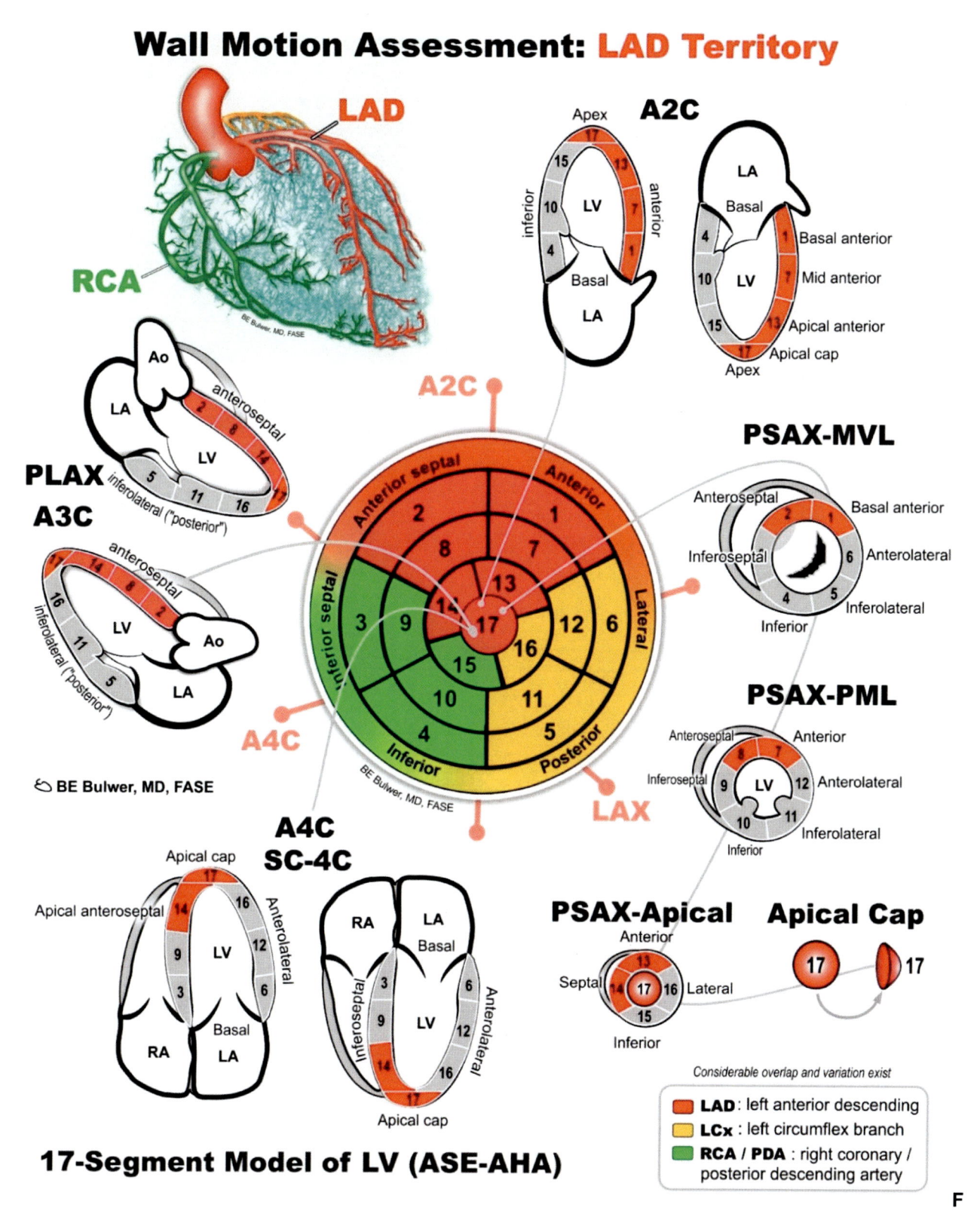

Fig. 56. Panoramic views of the polar or "bull's eye" plot of the left ventricular (LV) wall segments *(center)* **based on standards recommended by the American Society of Echocardiography (ASE).** These are color-coded to represent coronary artery supply as shown. The pattern of LV myocardial segments supplied by the **left anterior descending (LAD) coronary artery** is highlighted. Compare with Figs. 5-8, 55.

Coronary Artery Territories and Ischemic Patterns II

Wall Motion Assessment: LCx Territory

17-Segment Model of LV (ASE-AHA)

LAD: left anterior descending
LCx: left circumflex branch
RCA / PDA: right coronary / posterior descending artery

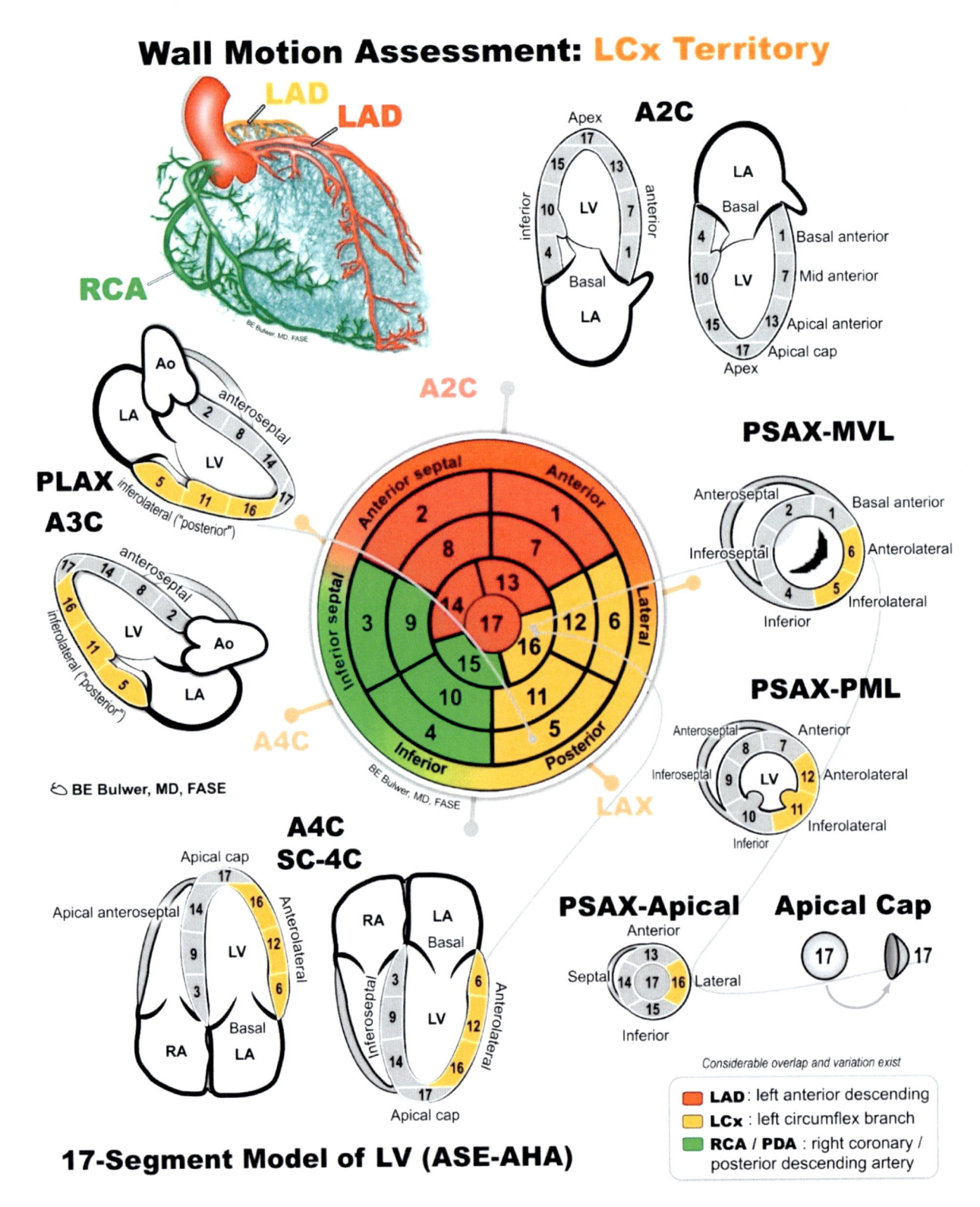

Considerable overlap and variation exist

Fig. 57. Panoramic views of the polar or "bull's eye" plot of the left ventricular (LV) wall segments *(center)* based on standards recommended by the American Society of Echocardiography (ASE). These are color-coded to represent coronary artery supply as shown. The pattern of LV myocardial segments supplied by the **left circumflex (LCx) coronary artery** is highlighted. Compare with Figs. 5-8, 55.

Coronary Artery Territories and Ischemic Patterns III

Wall Motion Assessment: RCA Territory

17-Segment Model of LV (ASE-AHA)

Considerable overlap and variation exist

- **LAD**: left anterior descending
- **LCx**: left circumflex branch
- **RCA / PDA**: right coronary / posterior descending artery

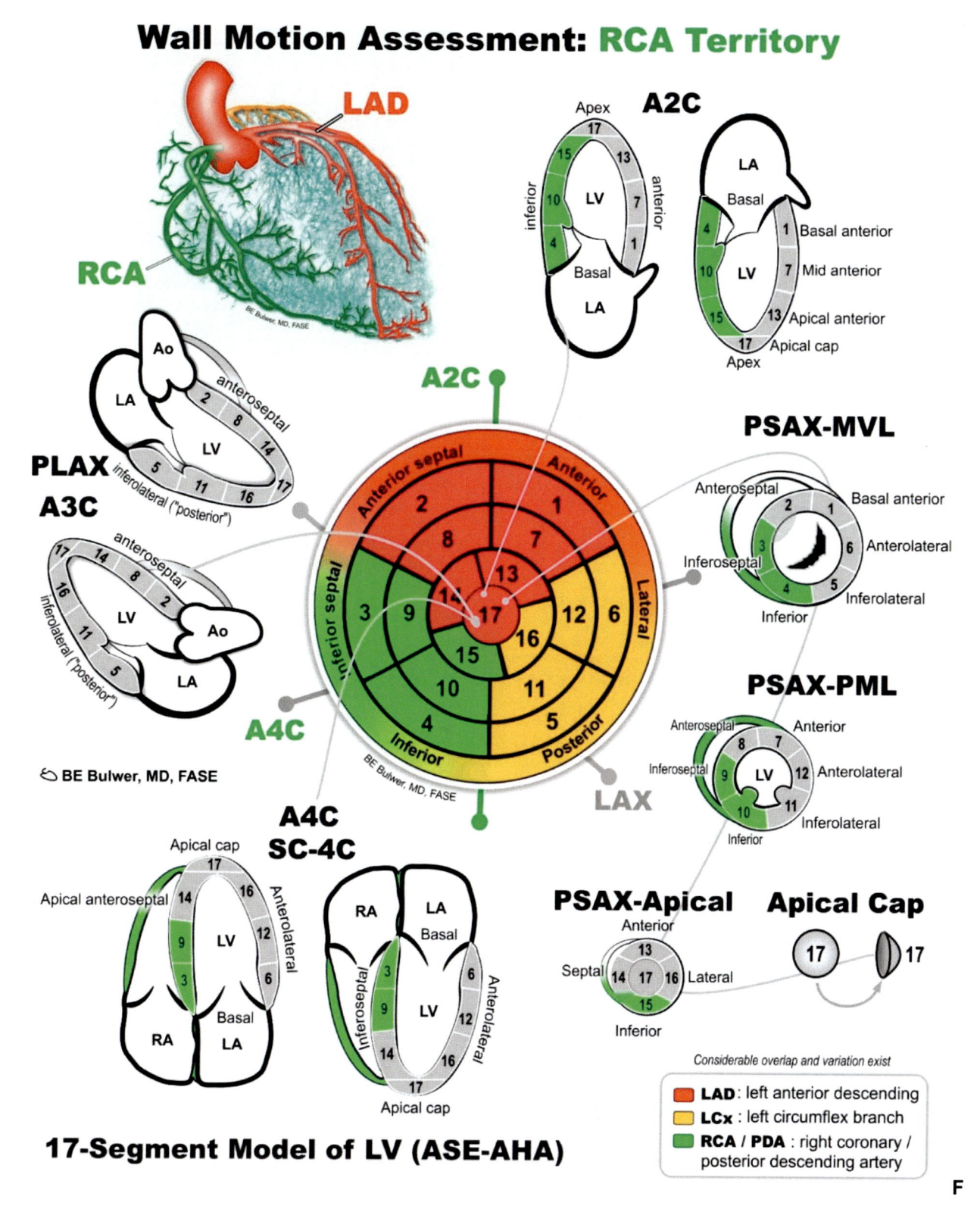

Fig. 58. **Panoramic views of the polar or "bull's eye" plot of the left ventricular (LV) wall segments *(center)* based on standards recommended by the American Society of Echocardiography (ASE).** These are color-coded to represent coronary artery supply as shown. The pattern of LV myocardial segments supplied by the **right coronary artery (RCA)** is highlighted. Compare with Figs. 5-8, 55.

F

Global and Regional Longitudinal Strain

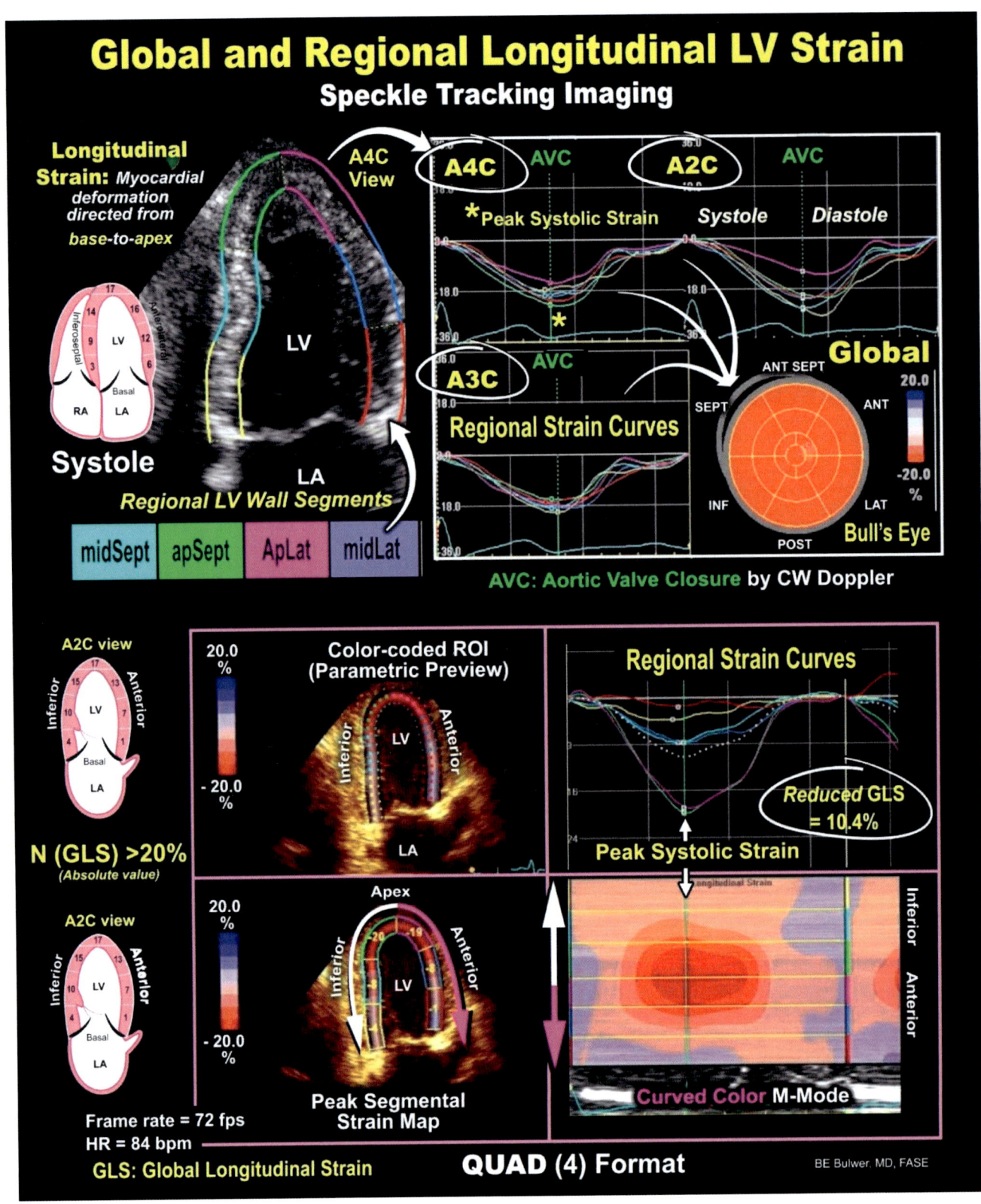

Fig. 59. **Myocardial strain imaging by speckle tracking echocardiography (STE).** Global longitudinal strain of the left ventricular myocardium on the apical four-chamber (A4C) *(upper panels)* and two-chamber (A2C) view *(lower panels)*. The "quad format" below shows four complementary parametric displays: (i) color-coded region of interest, (ii) segmental or regional strain curves, (iii) peak segmental strain, and (iv) curved anatomical color M-mode display of peak systolic strains. **Compare with Figs. 37-40, 47-55.**

Global Strain, Dyssynchrony, and Resynchronization

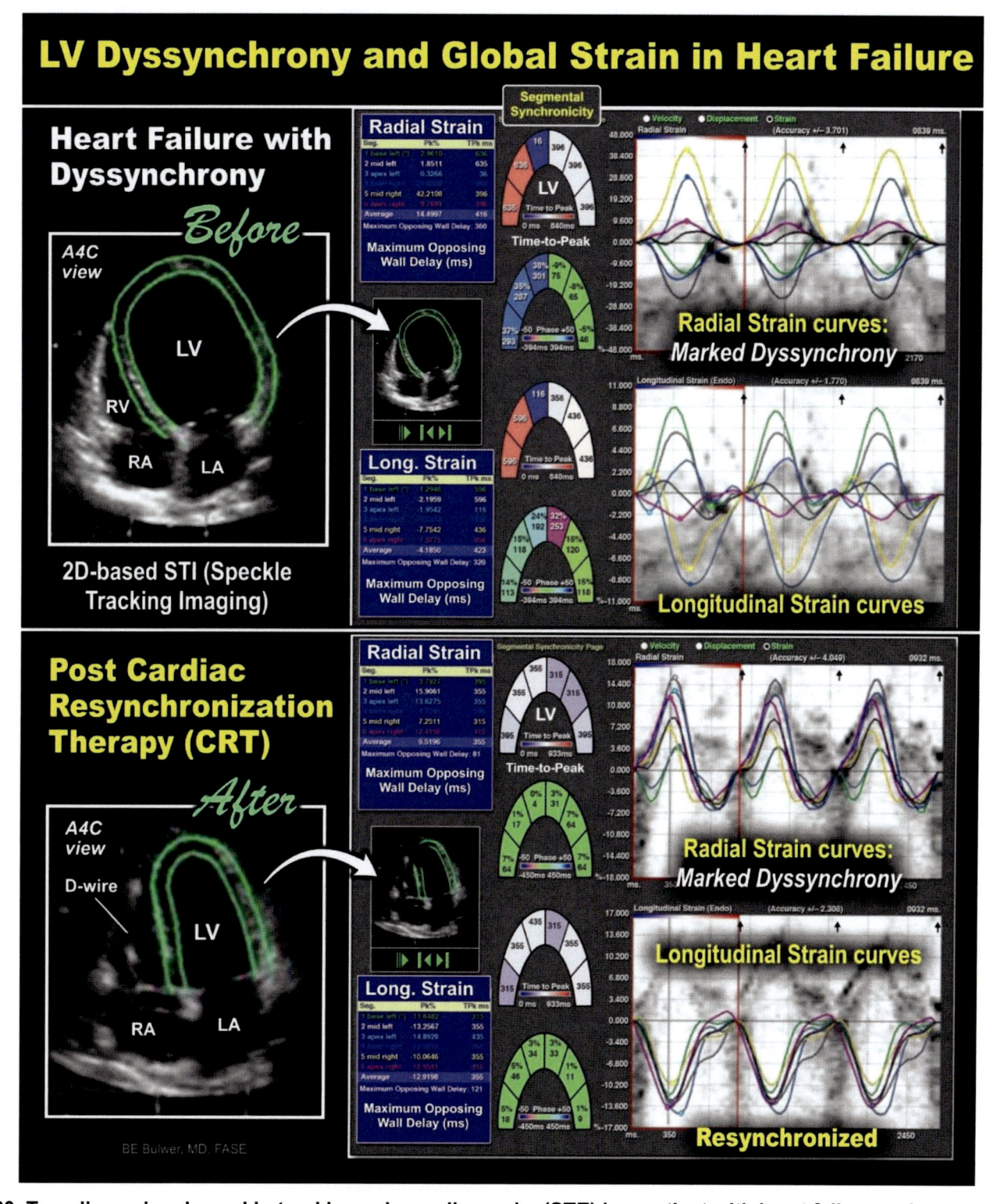

Fig. 60. Two-dimensional speckle-tracking echocardiography (STE) in a patient with heart failure and dyssynchrony before *(above)* and after cardiac resynchronization therapy and defibrillator (CRT-D) implantation *(below)*. The numerical values and labels on left ventricular (LV) segments *(center)* and curves *(right panels)* represent both the timing and magnitude of peak radial and longitudinal strains. The mid panels, a measure of interventricular dyssynchrony (impaired timing of LV wall contractions) indicate time-to-peak strain in 12 LV segments. Note the impact and improvement of these measures following CRT in the same patient.

Regional Wall Motion Assessment

Regional Wall Motion Assessment

Semiquantitative / Quantitative: by 2-D and 3-D Echocardiography

1. Acquire and Record Video Loops using the recommended TTE Echo Exam Protocol.
2. Use 16- or 17-Segment ASE/AHA/ACC LV Segmentation Model and Correlate with Coronary Artery Territory.

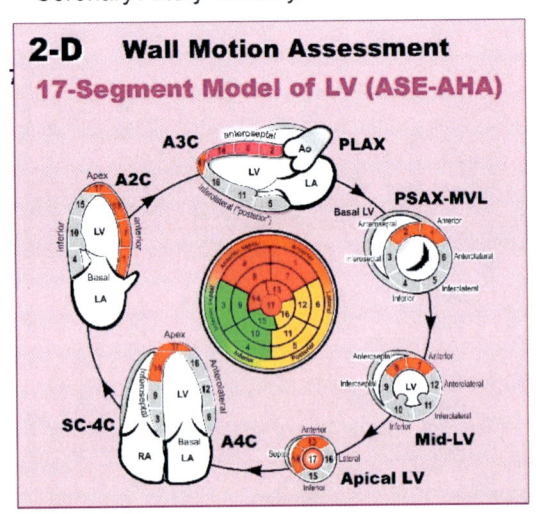

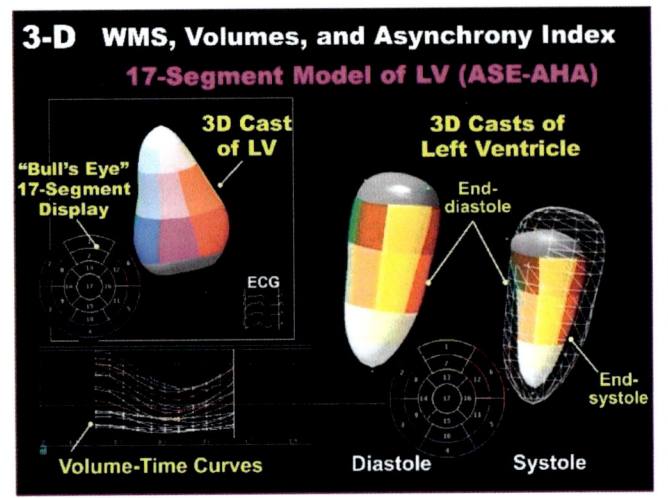

2-D Wall Motion Assessment — 17-Segment Model of LV (ASE-AHA)

3-D WMS, Volumes, and Asynchrony Index — 17-Segment Model of LV (ASE-AHA)

3. Observe Systolic LV Wall Motion in each view (Video loop) and score each segment, with special focus on: **A. Endocardial Motion (Squeeze)**, and **B. Wall Thickening**.

WALL MOTION SCORE Parameters
- A. Endocardial Motion
- B. Wall Thickening

Ensure Optimal Endocardial Border Visualiztion:
- Endocardium/Sub-endocardial layers of the myocardium contract to a greater degree (30% -70% more) than the outer sub-epicardial layers.

4. Record Wall Motion Scores and WMS Index (Automated calculation).
5. Avoid foreshortened LV views and beware pseudodyskinesis.

Wall Motion Score (WMS)

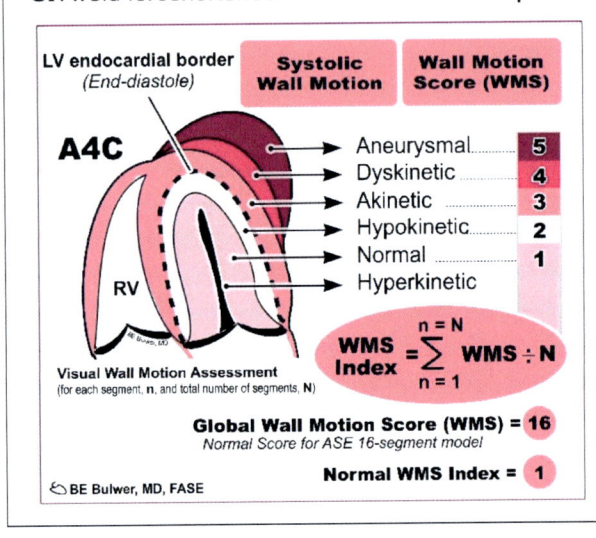

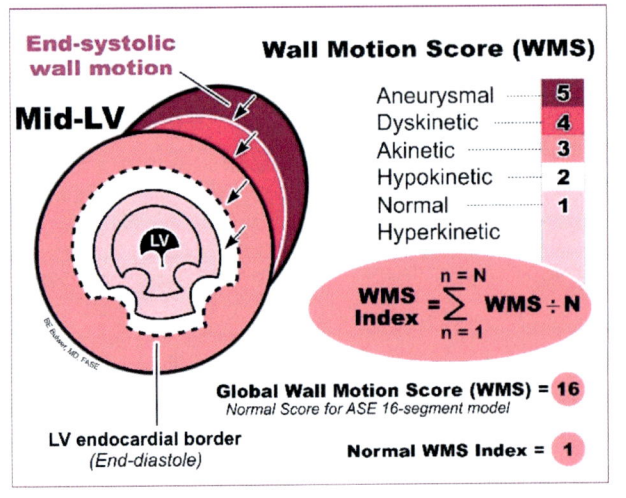

Wall Motion	Score
Aneurysmal	5
Dyskinetic	4
Akinetic	3
Hypokinetic	2
Normal	1
Hyperkinetic	

$$\text{WMS Index} = \sum_{n=1}^{n=N} \text{WMS} \div N$$

Global Wall Motion Score (WMS) = 16
Normal Score for ASE 16-segment model
Normal WMS Index = 1

Fig 61. Left ventricular (LV) regional wall motion can assessed by two-dimensional (2D) or three-dimensional (3D) echocardiography (Steps 1 to 5). Coronary artery disease is a leading cause of regional wall motion abnormality. See Figs. 28-60.

Post-Infarction LV Remodeling and Volume Changes

Post-Infarction Left Ventricular Remodeling

Acute Infarction — papillary muscle, Ao, LA, LV, mitral valve, Infarct territory

Infarct Expansion — LV, MR jet, Modified left parasternal long-axis perspective

Global LV Remodeling — LV

	Hours	Days to Months	Months to Years
RWMA	+	+	+
LV Diameters	N	+	+ +
LV Volumes	N	+	+ +
LV Mass	N	+	+ +
MR	− / +	+	+ +

LA: left atrium, LV: left ventricle, MR: mitral regurgitation, RWMA: regional wall motion abnormality

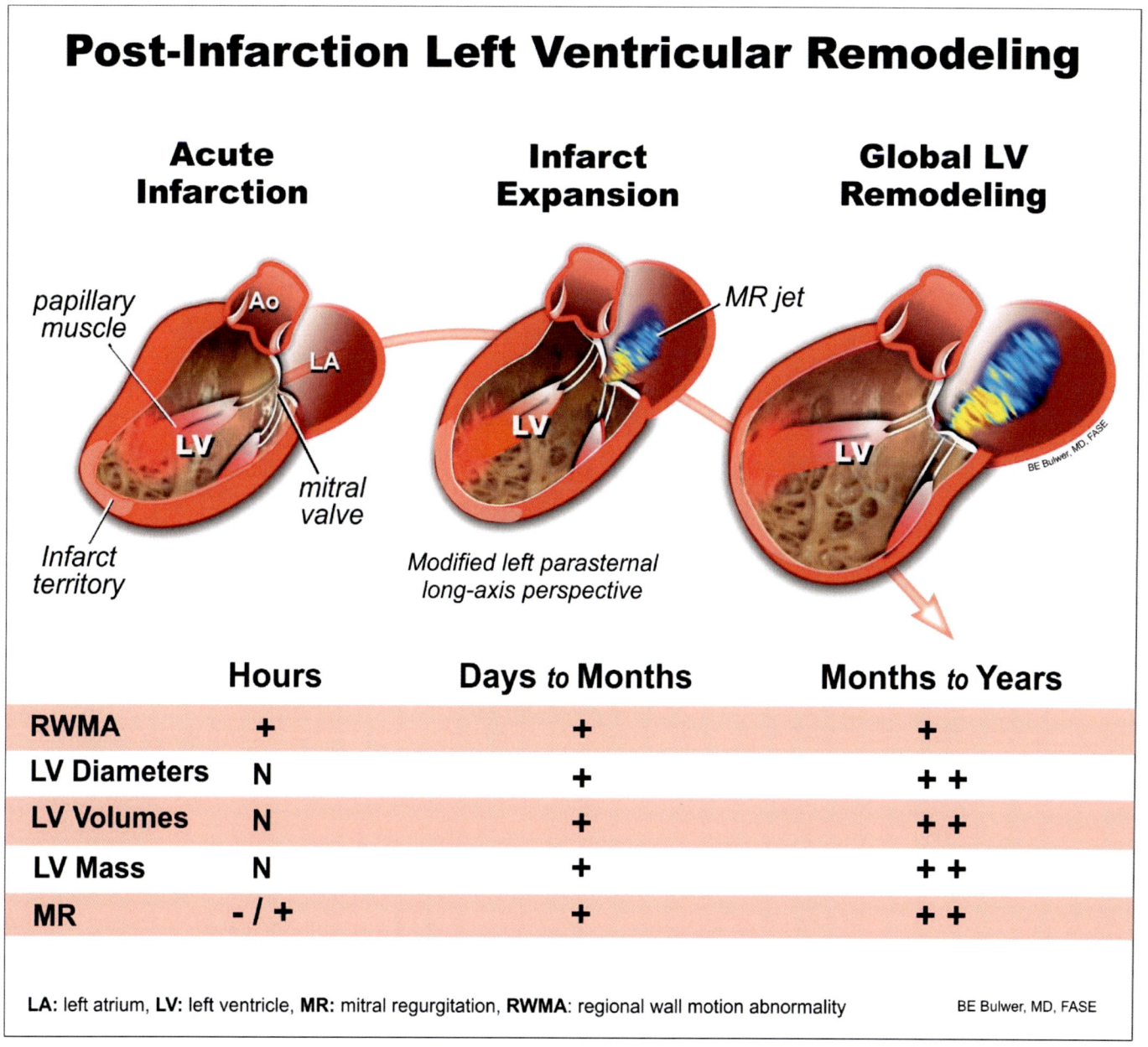

BE Bulwer, MD, FASE

Fig 62. Qualitative and quantitative measures of global left ventricular (LV) systolic function in patients with coronary artery disease. Note the impact of time on regional wall motion abnormalities (RWMA) and other indices of ventricular function post-myocardial infarction.

Coronary Artery Supply to the RIGHT VENTRICLE – RV

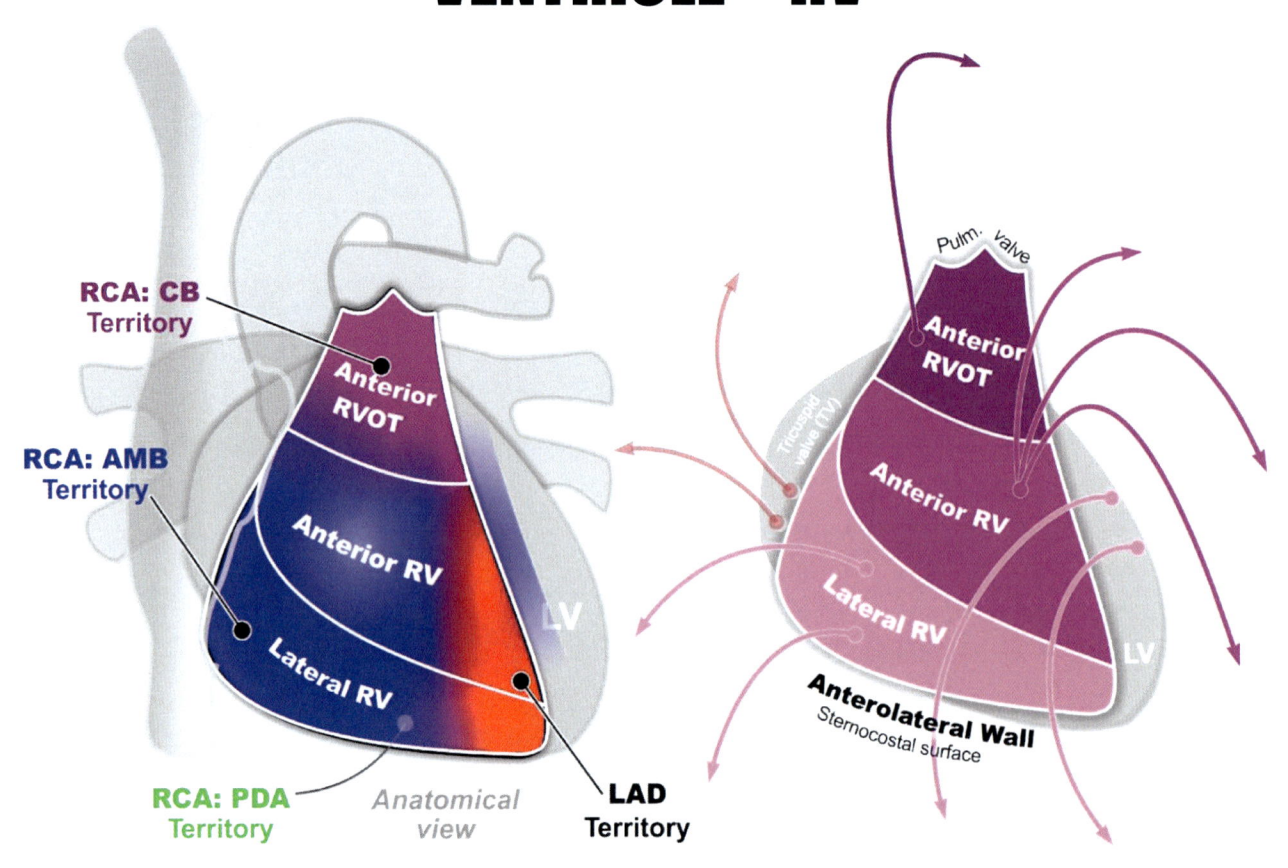

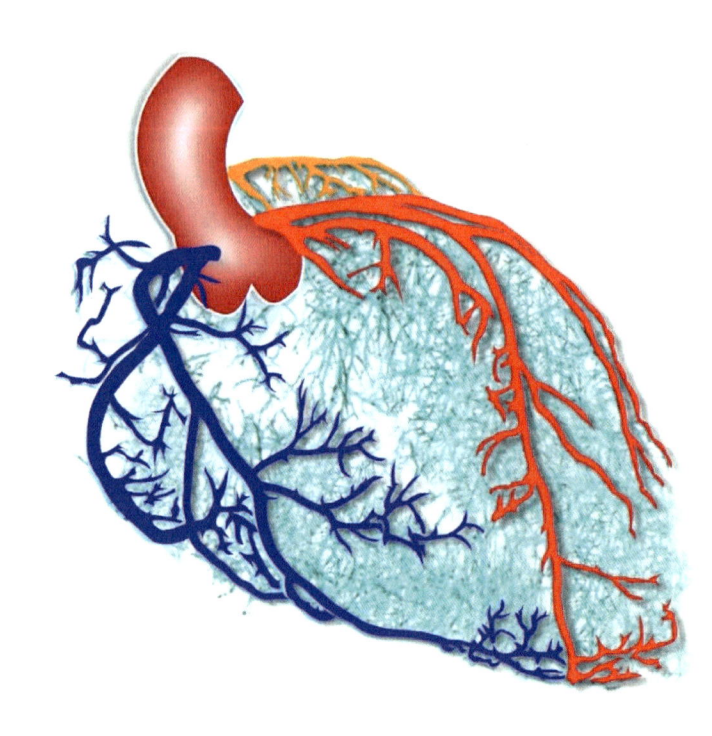

Coronary Artery Anatomy and the Right Ventricle

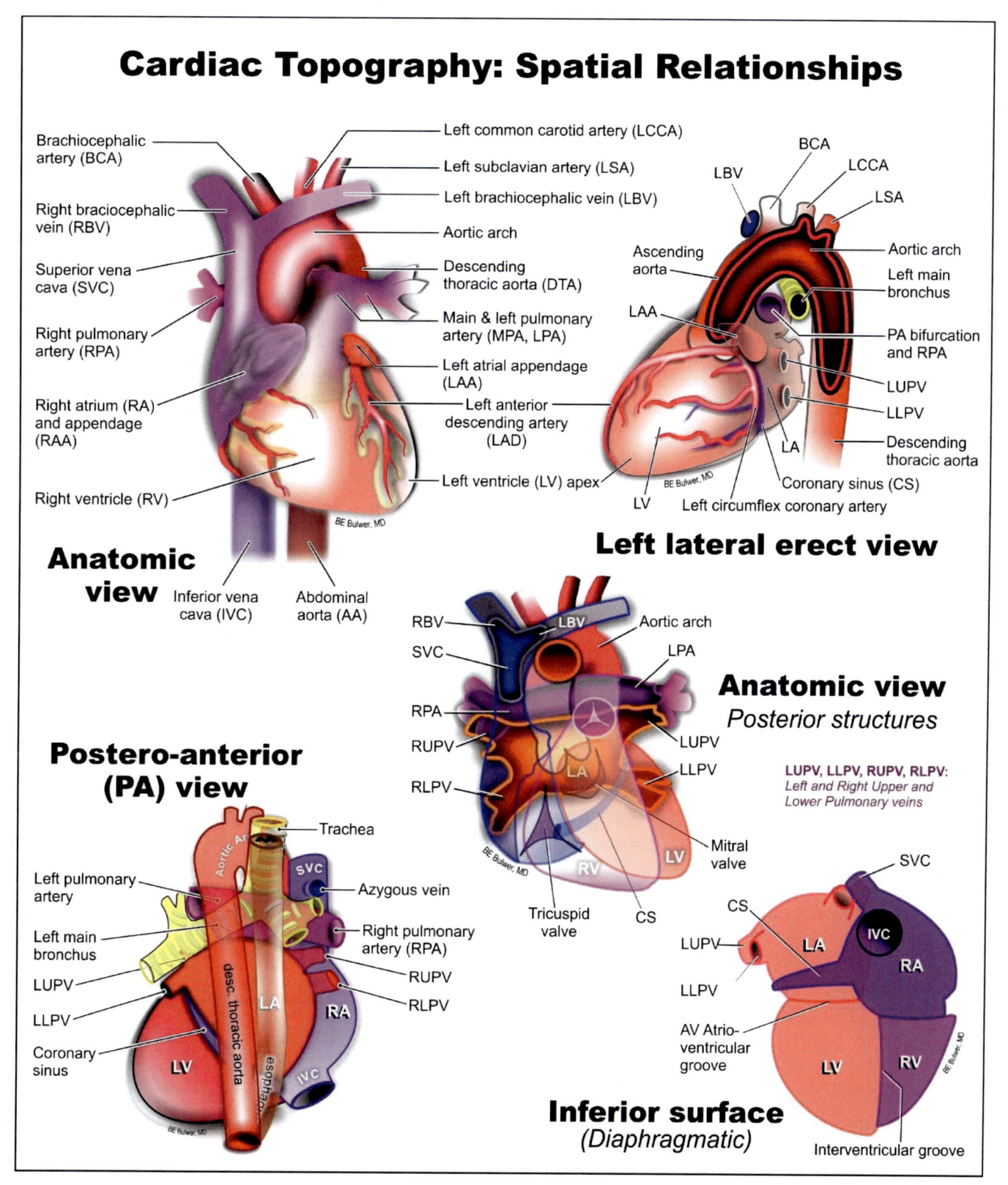

Fig. 63. Three-dimensional anatomical perspectives of the right ventricle. Note the orientation and topographical relationships of the right ventricle (RV) relative to the other cardiac chambers and major vessels, including the epicardial coronary arteries.

3D Echocardiographic Anatomy

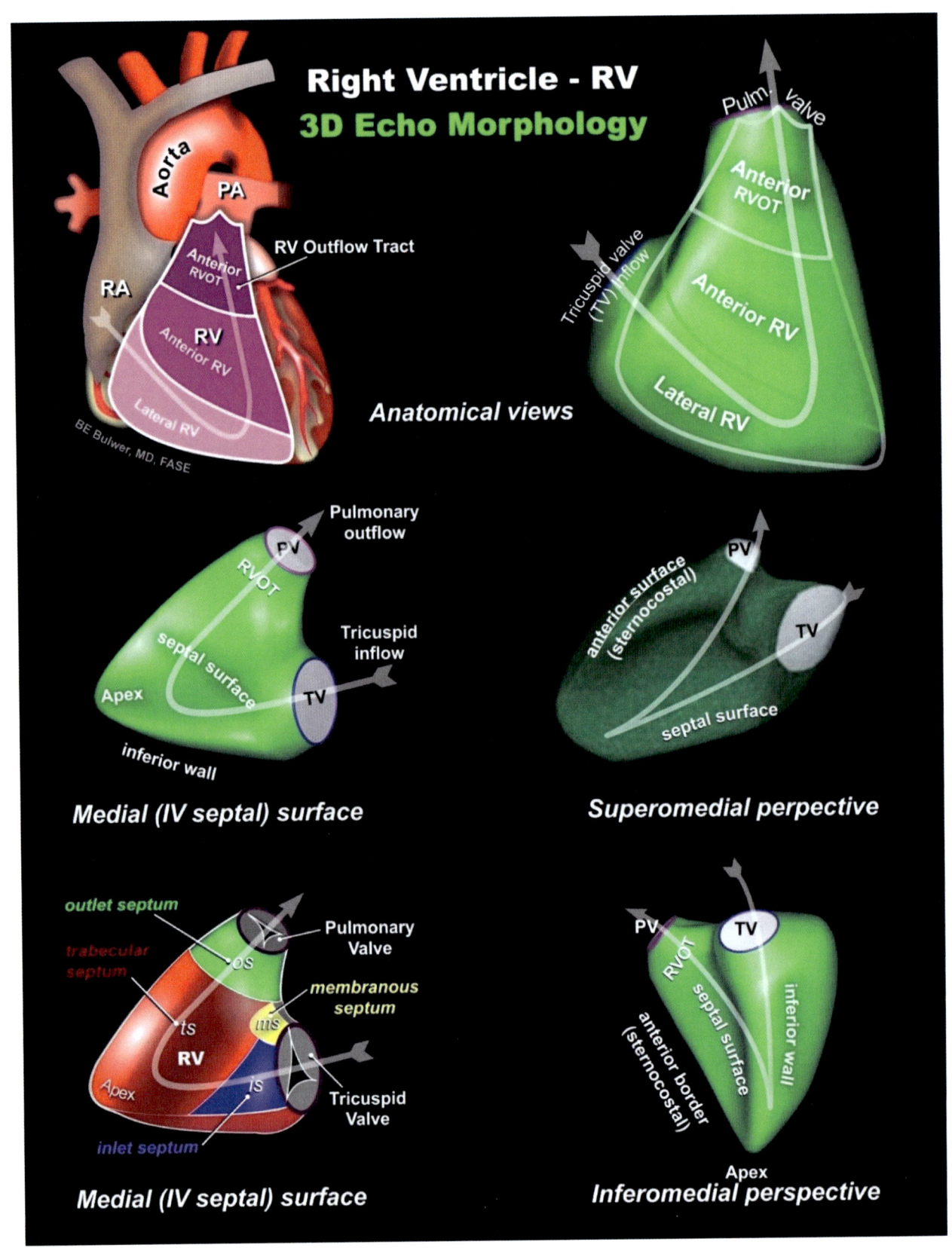

Fig. 64. **Three-dimensional (3D) transthoracic echocardiographic (3D-TTE) perspectives showing the orientation and morphology of the right ventricle (RV).** These 3D volumetric casts of the RV were reconstructed and rendered using proprietary software. Note the irregular crescentic shape of the RV compared to the LV.

2D Echo Assessment of the Right Ventricle I

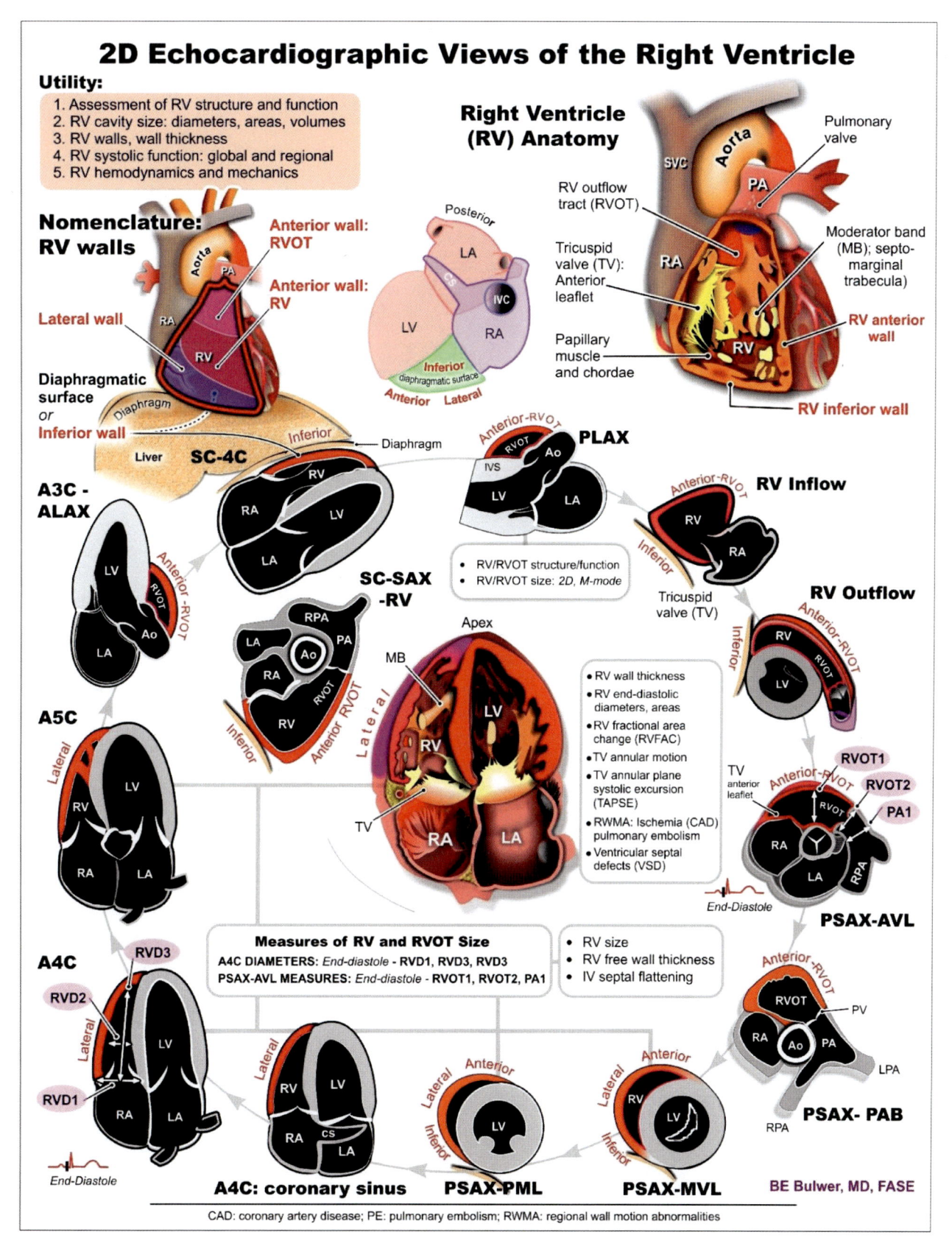

Fig. 65. Cross-sectional views of the right ventricle (RV) and RV walls. Note the nomenclature of the RV walls, the nomenclature of the RV segments and their corresponding coronary artery supply (Figs. 64-75).

2D Echo Assessment of the Right Ventricle II

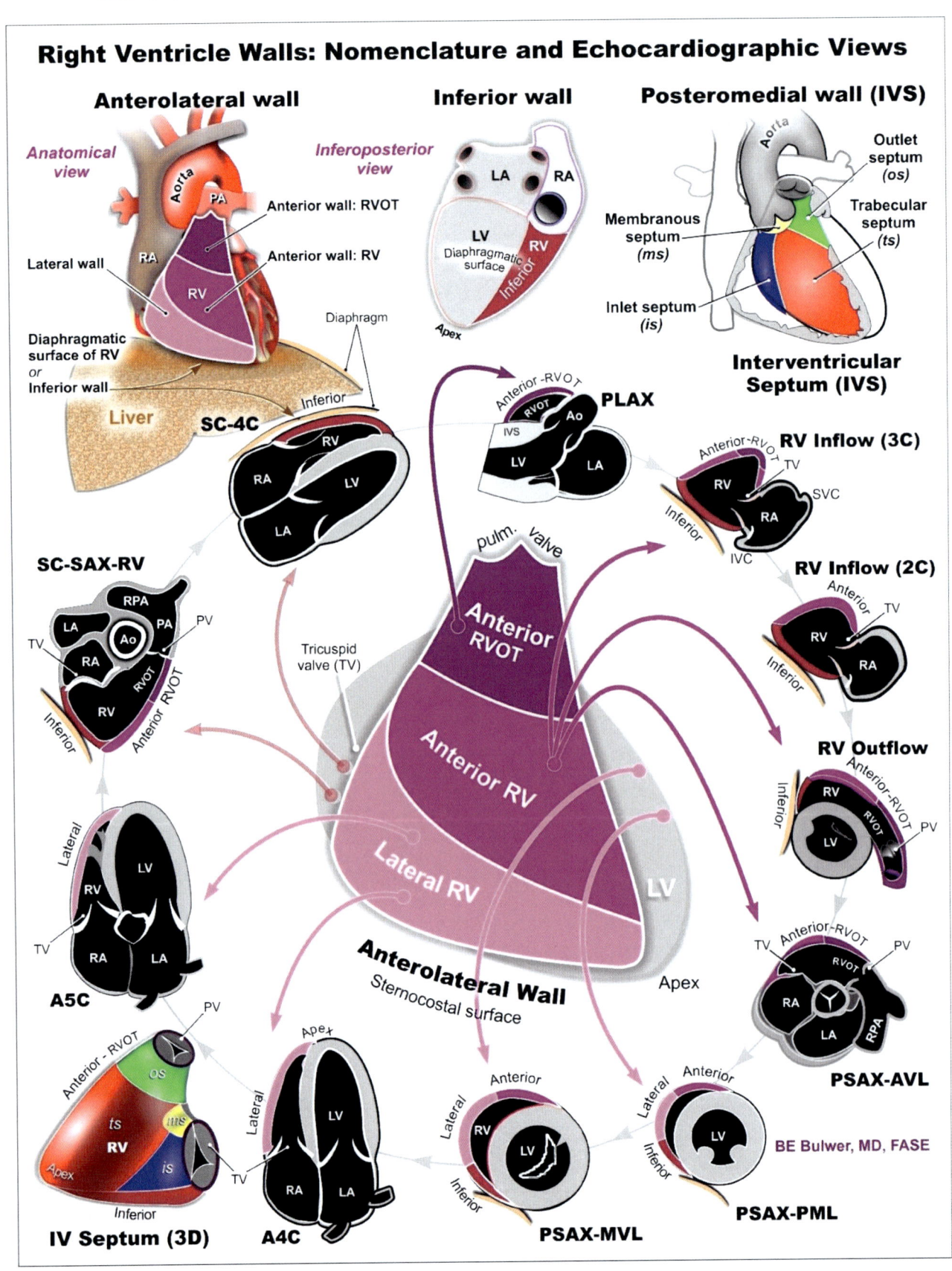

Fig. 66. Nomenclature of the right ventricular (RV) wall, segments and their corresponding coronary artery supply (Figs. 64-75).

2D Echo Assessment of the Right Ventricle III

Echo Assessment of Right Ventricular (RV) Size

1. RV Linear Dimensions - Inflow

- A4C view - RV focused
- End-diastolic measurements

RVD1: Basal RV linear dimension - basal one third of RV inflow
RVD2: Mid-cavity RV linear dimension - the transverse RV diameter in the middle third of RV inflow (half-way point)

Advantages
- Technical ease
- Basic
- Quick
- Much published data

Limitations
- RV shape irregular, and size easy to underestimate - irregular shape
- RV linear dimensions affected by image aquisition technique, i.e. skill-operator dependent
- Echo Report should document imaging window used to perform measurements

2. RV Linear Dimensions - Outflow

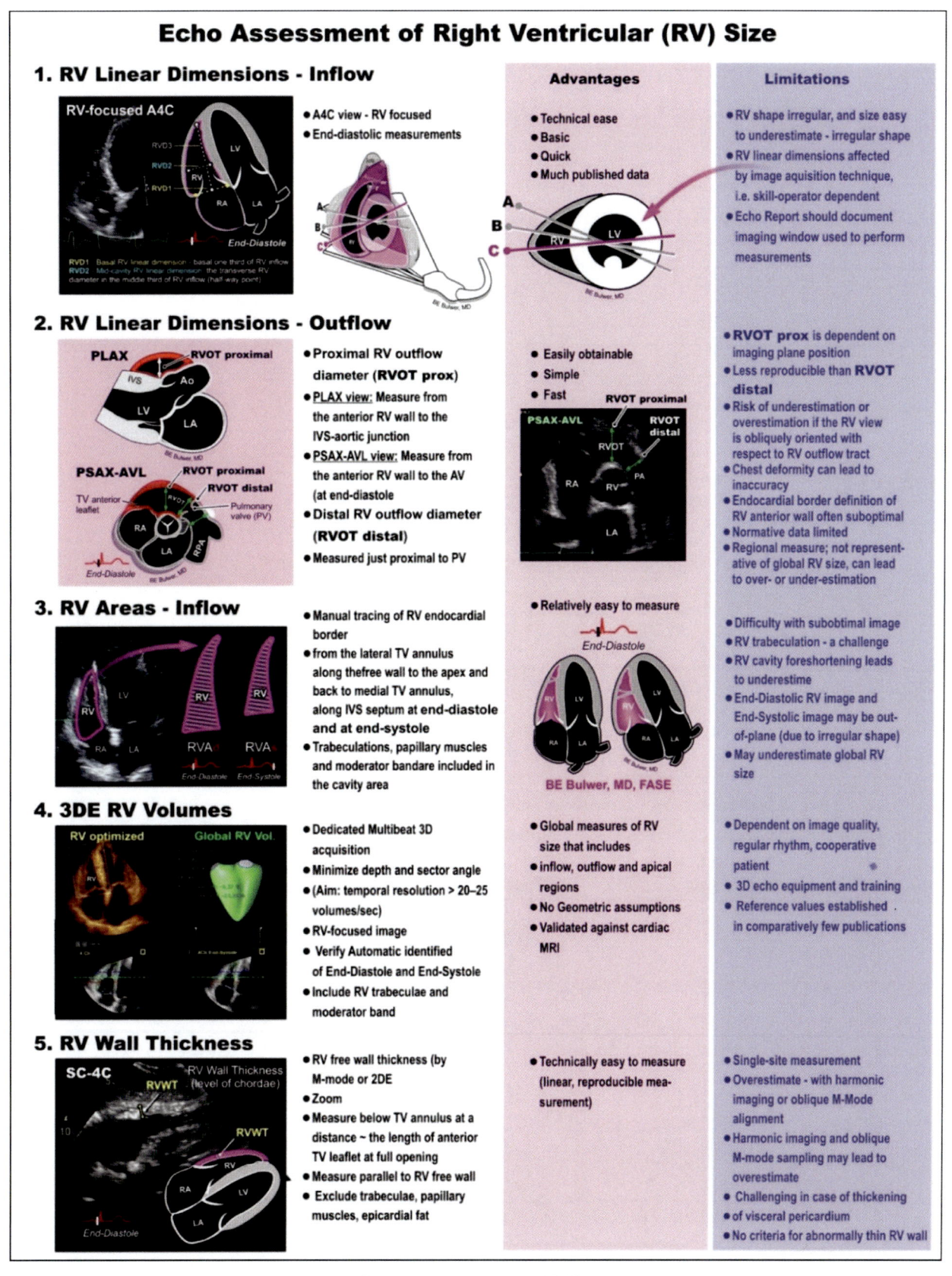

- Proximal RV outflow diameter (**RVOT prox**)
- **PLAX view:** Measure from the anterior RV wall to the IVS-aortic junction
- **PSAX-AVL view:** Measure from the anterior RV wall to the AV (at end-diastole
- Distal RV outflow diameter (**RVOT distal**)
- Measured just proximal to PV

Advantages
- Easily obtainable
- Simple
- Fast

Limitations
- **RVOT prox** is dependent on imaging plane position
- Less reproducible than **RVOT distal**
- Risk of underestimation or overestimation if the RV view is obliquely oriented with respect to RV outflow tract
- Chest deformity can lead to inaccuracy
- Endocardial border definition of RV anterior wall often suboptimal
- Normative data limited
- Regional measure; not represent-ative of global RV size, can lead to over- or under-estimation

3. RV Areas - Inflow

- Manual tracing of RV endocardial border
- from the lateral TV annulus along the free wall to the apex and back to medial TV annulus, along IVS septum at end-diastole and at end-systole
- Trabeculations, papillary muscles and moderator band are included in the cavity area

Advantages
- Relatively easy to measure

Limitations
- Difficulty with suboptimal image
- RV trabeculation - a challenge
- RV cavity foreshortening leads to underestime
- End-Diastolic RV image and End-Systolic image may be out-of-plane (due to irregular shape)
- May underestimate global RV size

4. 3DE RV Volumes

- Dedicated Multibeat 3D acquisition
- Minimize depth and sector angle
- (Aim: temporal resolution > 20–25 volumes/sec)
- RV-focused image
- Verify Automatic identified of End-Diastole and End-Systole
- Include RV trabeculae and moderator band

Advantages
- Global measures of RV size that includes
- inflow, outflow and apical regions
- No Geometric assumptions
- Validated against cardiac MRI

Limitations
- Dependent on image quality, regular rhythm, cooperative patient
- 3D echo equipment and training
- Reference values established in comparatively few publications

5. RV Wall Thickness

- RV free wall thickness (by M-mode or 2DE
- Zoom
- Measure below TV annulus at a distance ~ the length of anterior TV leaflet at full opening
- Measure parallel to RV free wall
- Exclude trabeculae, papillary muscles, epicardial fat

Advantages
- Technically easy to measure (linear, reproducible mea-surement)

Limitations
- Single-site measurement
- Overestimate - with harmonic imaging or oblique M-Mode alignment
- Harmonic imaging and oblique M-mode sampling may lead to overestimate
- Challenging in case of thickening of visceral pericardium
- No criteria for abnormally thin RV wall

Fig. 67. Echocardiographic assessment of the right ventricle (RV) is integral to the comprehensive assessment of coronary artery disease. This includes the assessment of RV linear dimensions, areas, and volumes. Compare with Figs. 61, 62.

2D Echo Assessment of the Right Ventricle IV

Echo Assessment of Right Ventricular (RV) Function II

1. Pulsed Tissue Doppler Imaging: S-Wave

Advantages
- Technically easy
- Reproducible
- Validation (with radionuclide Ejection Fraction -EF)
- Prognostic value

Limitations
- Angle dependent, therefore Optimize parallel alignment of TA (RV free wall) longitudinal shortening
- RV global function along longitudinal direction only
- Caution in utilizing this technique post:
  - thoracotomy,
  - pulmonary thromboendarterectomy or
  - heart transplantation

2. Color Tissue Doppler S-Wave

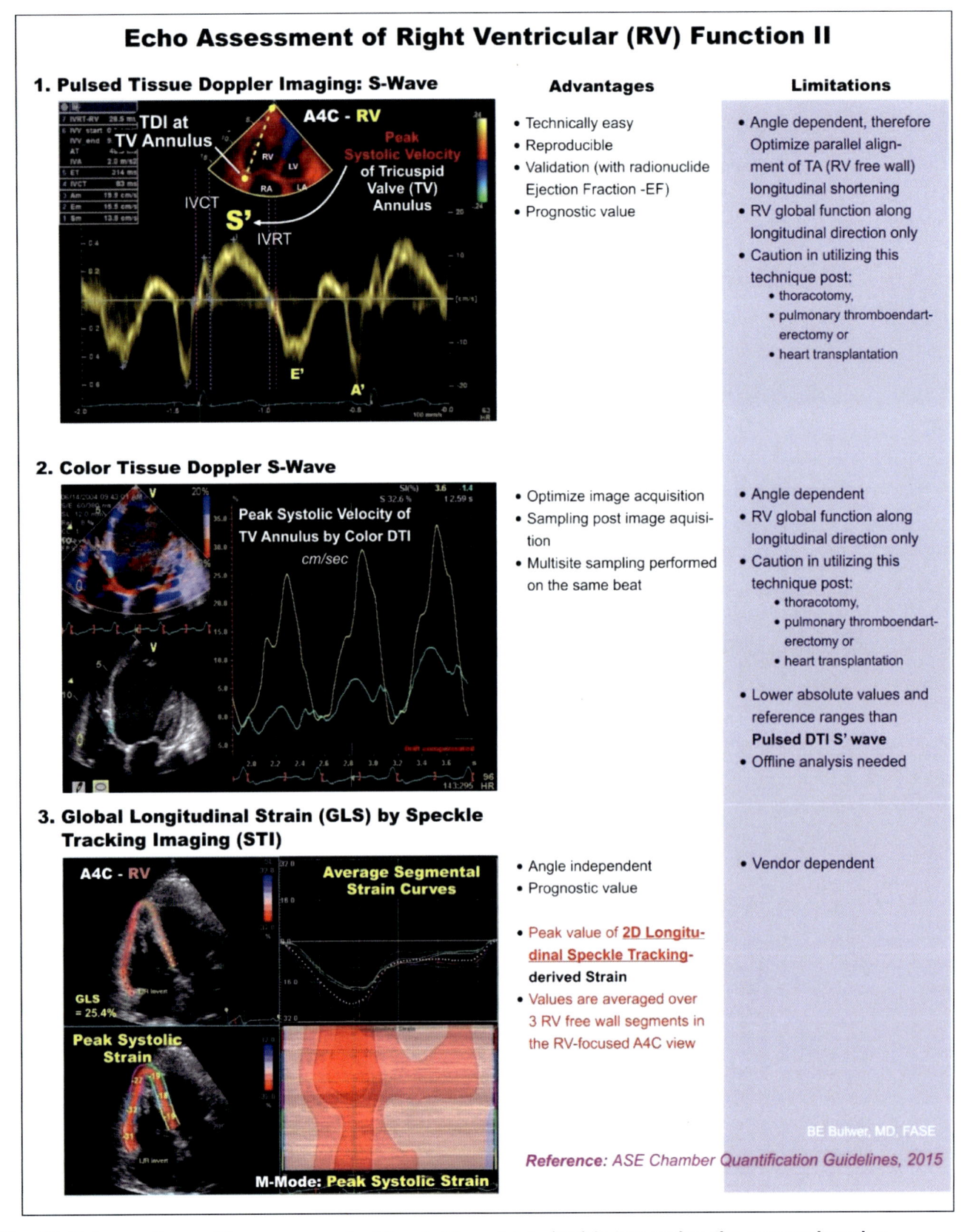

Advantages
- Optimize image acquisition
- Sampling post image aquisition
- Multisite sampling performed on the same beat

Limitations
- Angle dependent
- RV global function along longitudinal direction only
- Caution in utilizing this technique post:
  - thoracotomy,
  - pulmonary thromboendarterectomy or
  - heart transplantation
- Lower absolute values and reference ranges than **Pulsed DTI S' wave**
- Offline analysis needed

3. Global Longitudinal Strain (GLS) by Speckle Tracking Imaging (STI)

Advantages
- Angle independent
- Prognostic value
- Peak value of **2D Longitudinal Speckle Tracking-**derived Strain
- Values are averaged over 3 RV free wall segments in the RV-focused A4C view

Limitations
- Vendor dependent

Reference: ASE Chamber Quantification Guidelines, 2015

Fig. 68. Echocardiographic assessment of the right ventricle (RV) is integral to the comprehensive assessment of coronary artery disease. Assessment of the RV myocardium includes tissue Doppler imaging (TDI) and derived measures such as RV strain. Compare with Figs. 38-48.

Coronary Arteries Supply to the Right Ventricle I

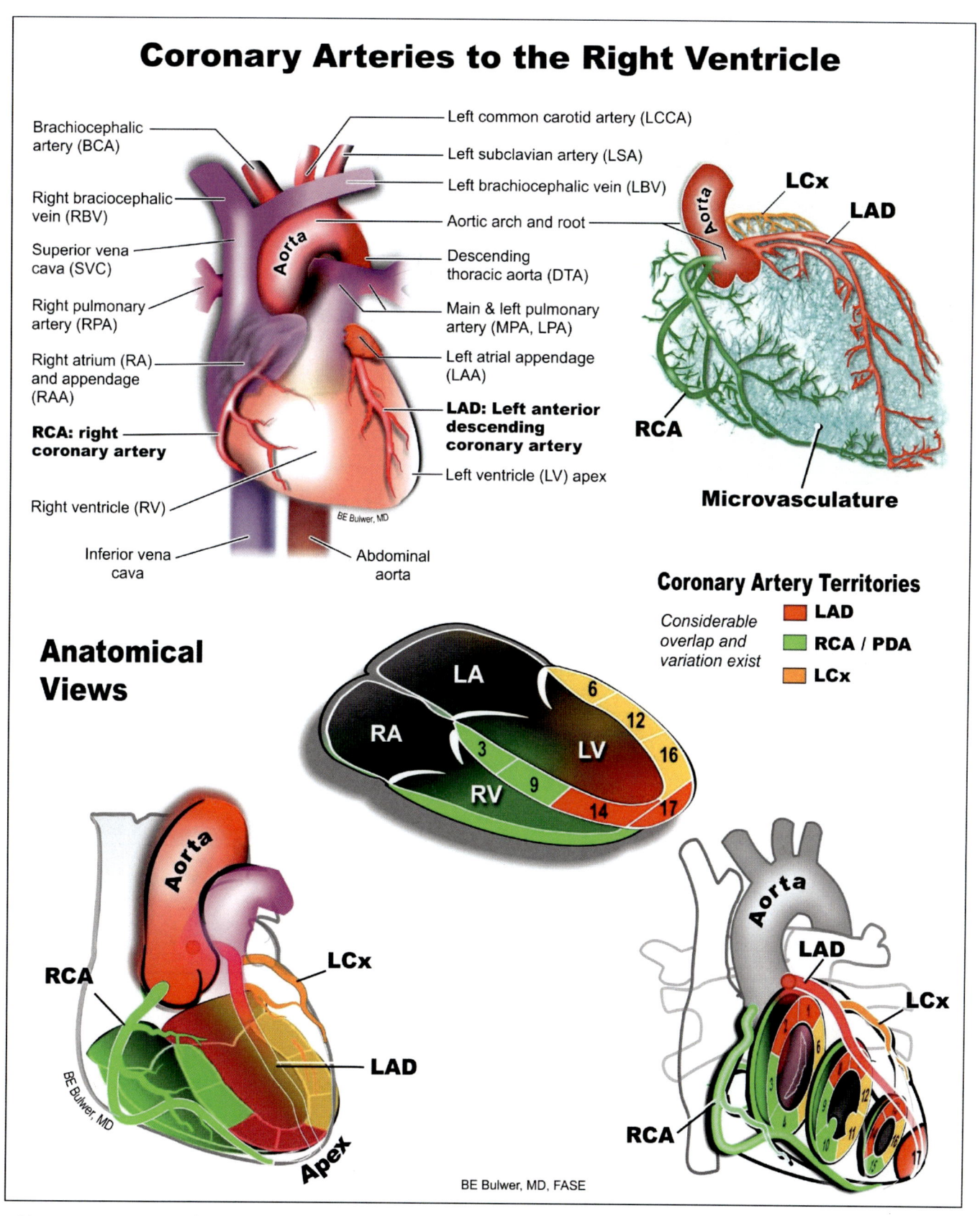

Fig 69. Anatomical view of the heart with focus on the right coronary artery (RCA) and ventricular territories supplied by the RCA. Correlate with Figs. 70-75.

Coronary Arteries Supply to the Right Ventricle II

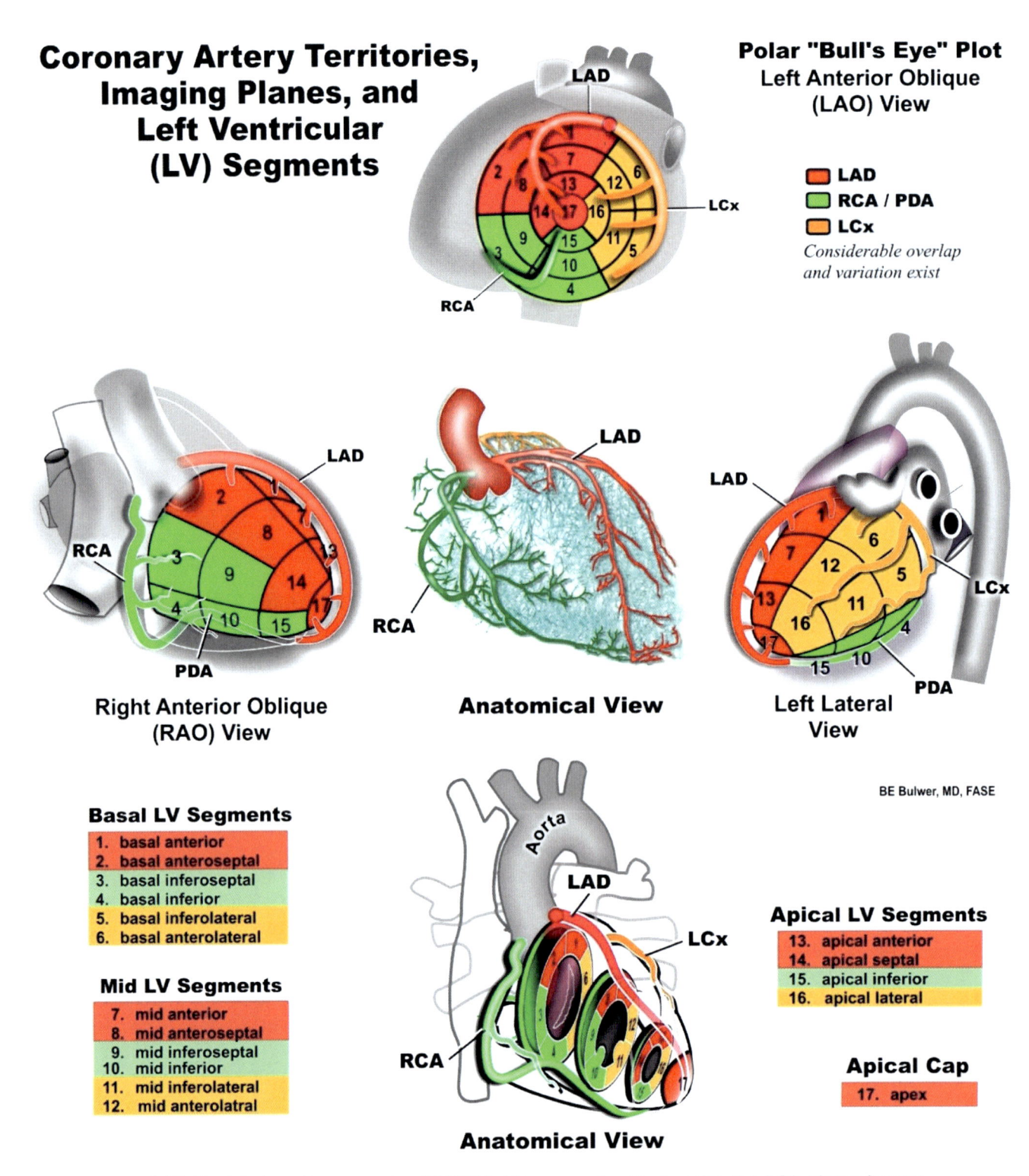

Coronary Artery Territories, Imaging Planes, and Left Ventricular (LV) Segments

Polar "Bull's Eye" Plot
Left Anterior Oblique (LAO) View

- LAD
- RCA / PDA
- LCx

Considerable overlap and variation exist

Right Anterior Oblique (RAO) View

Anatomical View

Left Lateral View

BE Bulwer, MD, FASE

Basal LV Segments
1. basal anterior
2. basal anteroseptal
3. basal inferoseptal
4. basal inferior
5. basal inferolateral
6. basal anterolateral

Mid LV Segments
7. mid anterior
8. mid anteroseptal
9. mid inferoseptal
10. mid inferior
11. mid inferolateral
12. mid anterolatral

Apical LV Segments
13. apical anterior
14. apical septal
15. apical inferior
16. apical lateral

Apical Cap
17. apex

Anatomical View

LAD, left anterior descending coronary artery; **RCA/PDA**, right coronary and posteior descending artery; **LCA**, left circumflex artery

Fig. 70. **Panoramic views of the heart showing the major epicardial coronary arteries and their corresponding ventricular territories.** Correlate with Figs. 71-75.

Coronary Arteries Supply to the Right Ventricle III

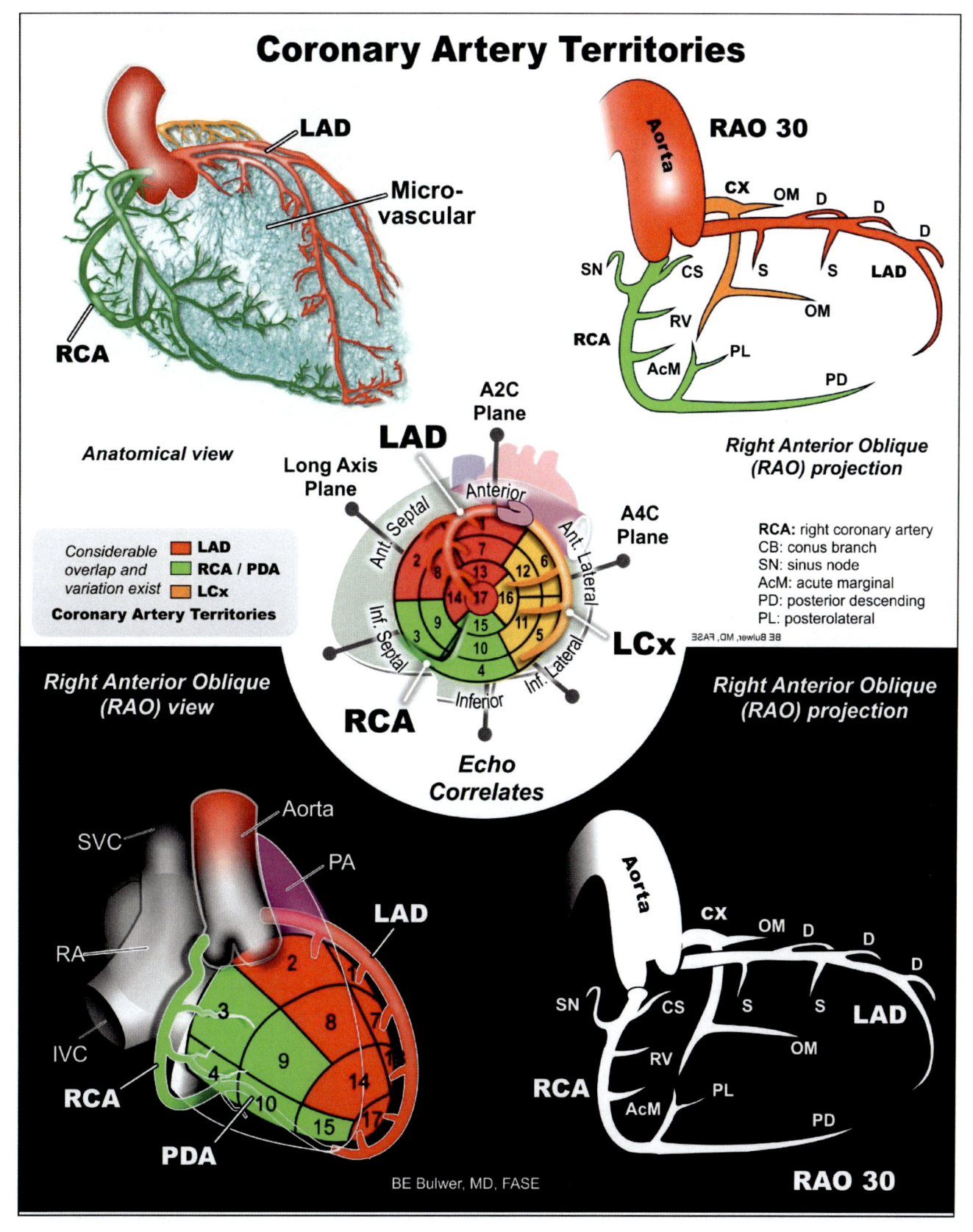

Fig. 71. Projections of coronary artery anatomy and ventricular segments, with focus on the right coronary artery (RCA). Correlate with Figs. 70-75.

Coronary Arteries Supply to the Right Ventricle IV

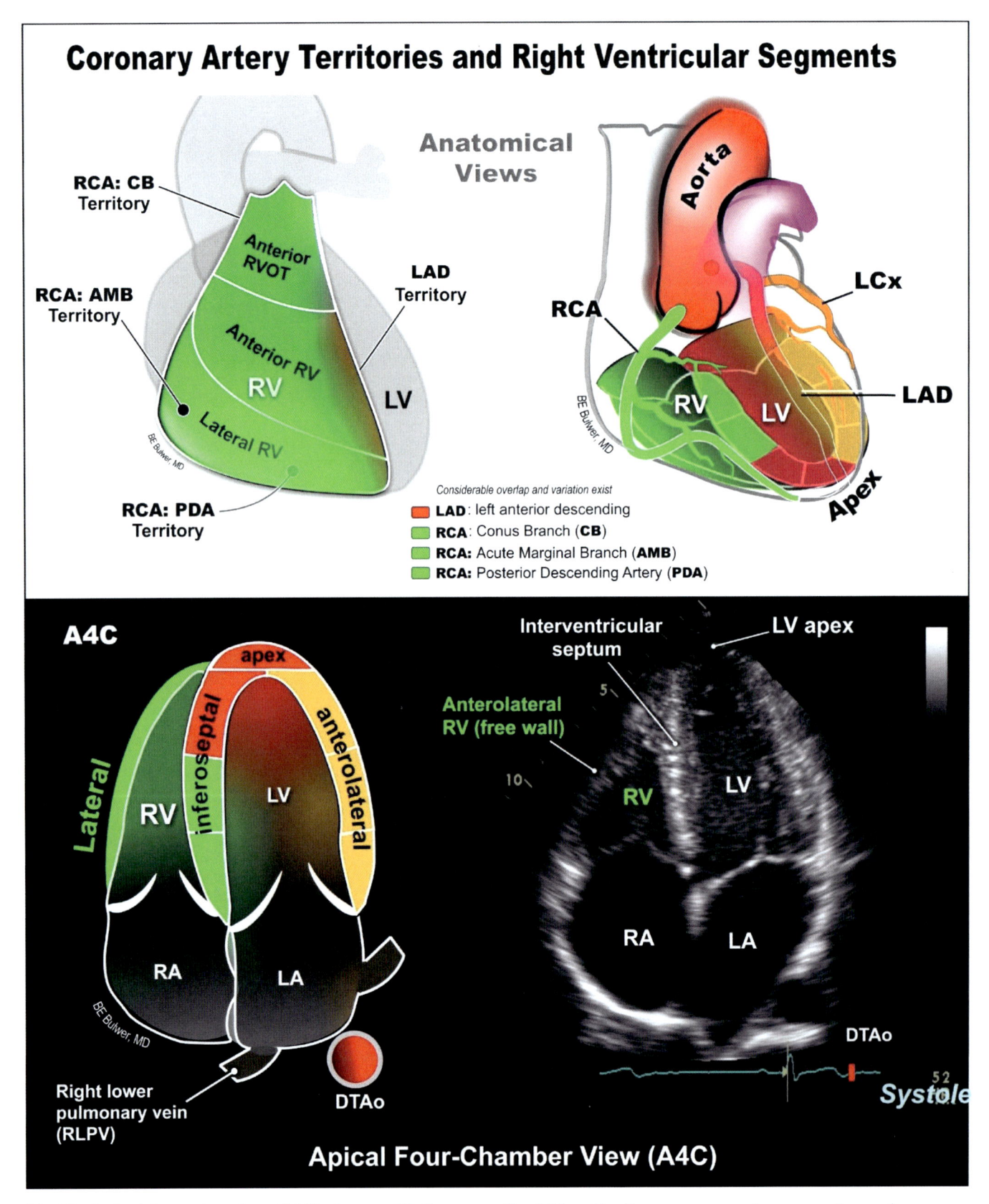

Fig 72. Apical four-chamber (A4C) views with focus on the RV walls, its coronary artery supply, and relationship to the LV. Most of the supply the RV free wall is through the right coronary (RCA). Compare with Figs. 73-75.

Coronary Arteries Supply to the Right Ventricle V

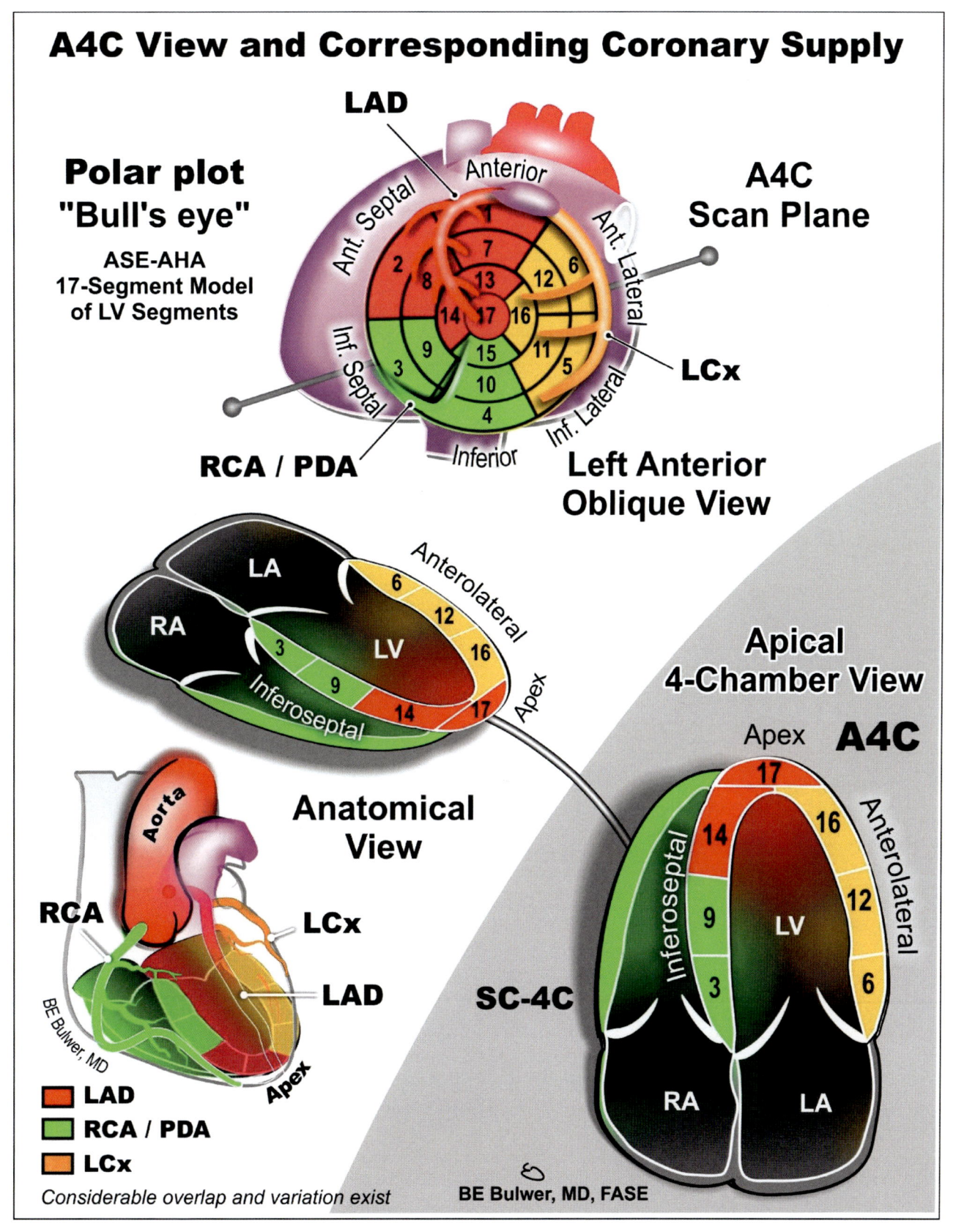

Fig 73. Panoramic perspectives of the apical four-chamber (A4C) view, the right ventricular (RV) walls and their coronary artery supply.

Coronary Arteries Supply to the Right Ventricle VI

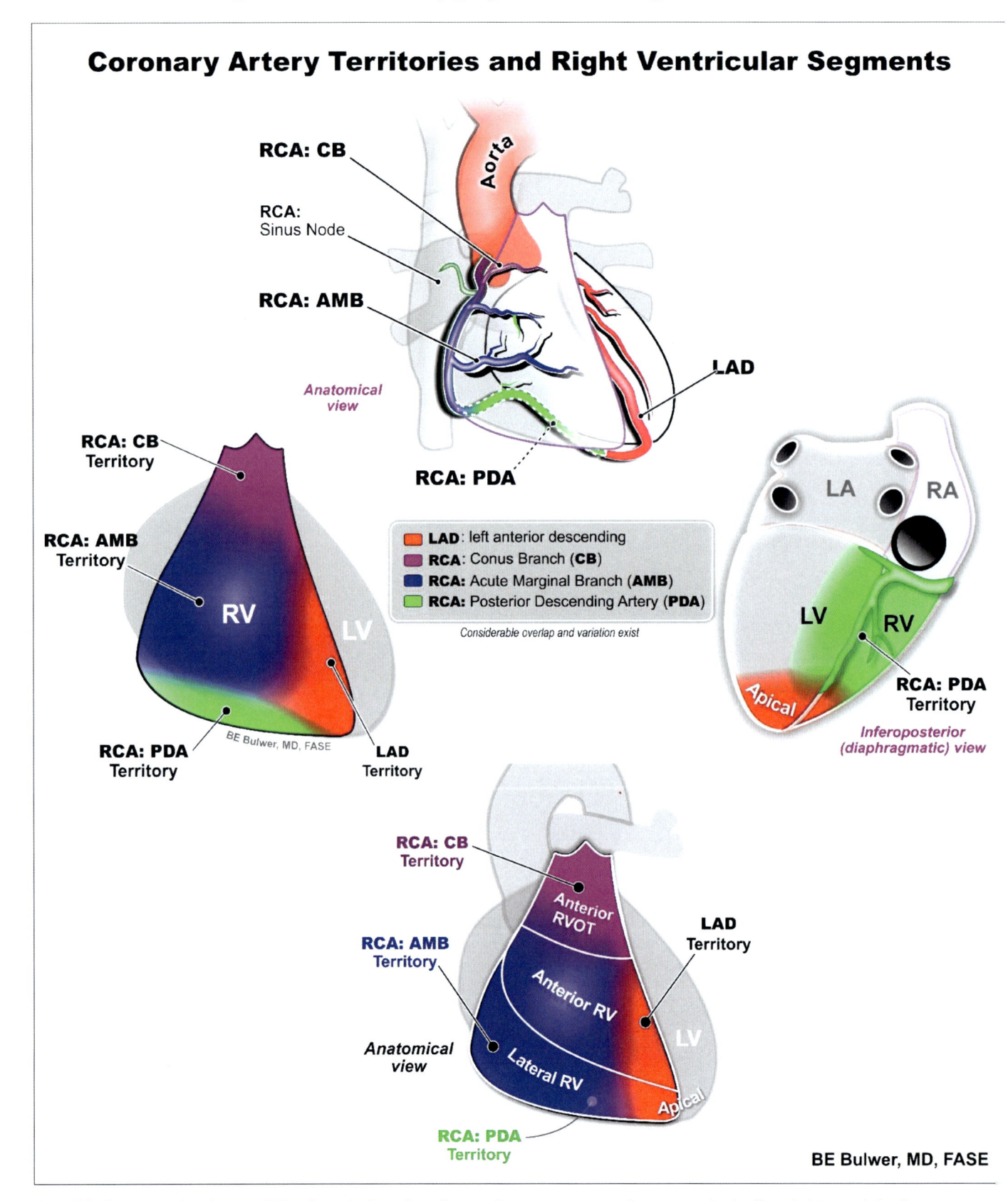

Fig. 74. Panoramic views of the heart showing the major coronary artery supply to the right ventricular walls. Compare with Figs. 69-75.

Coronary Arteries Supply to the Right Ventricle VII

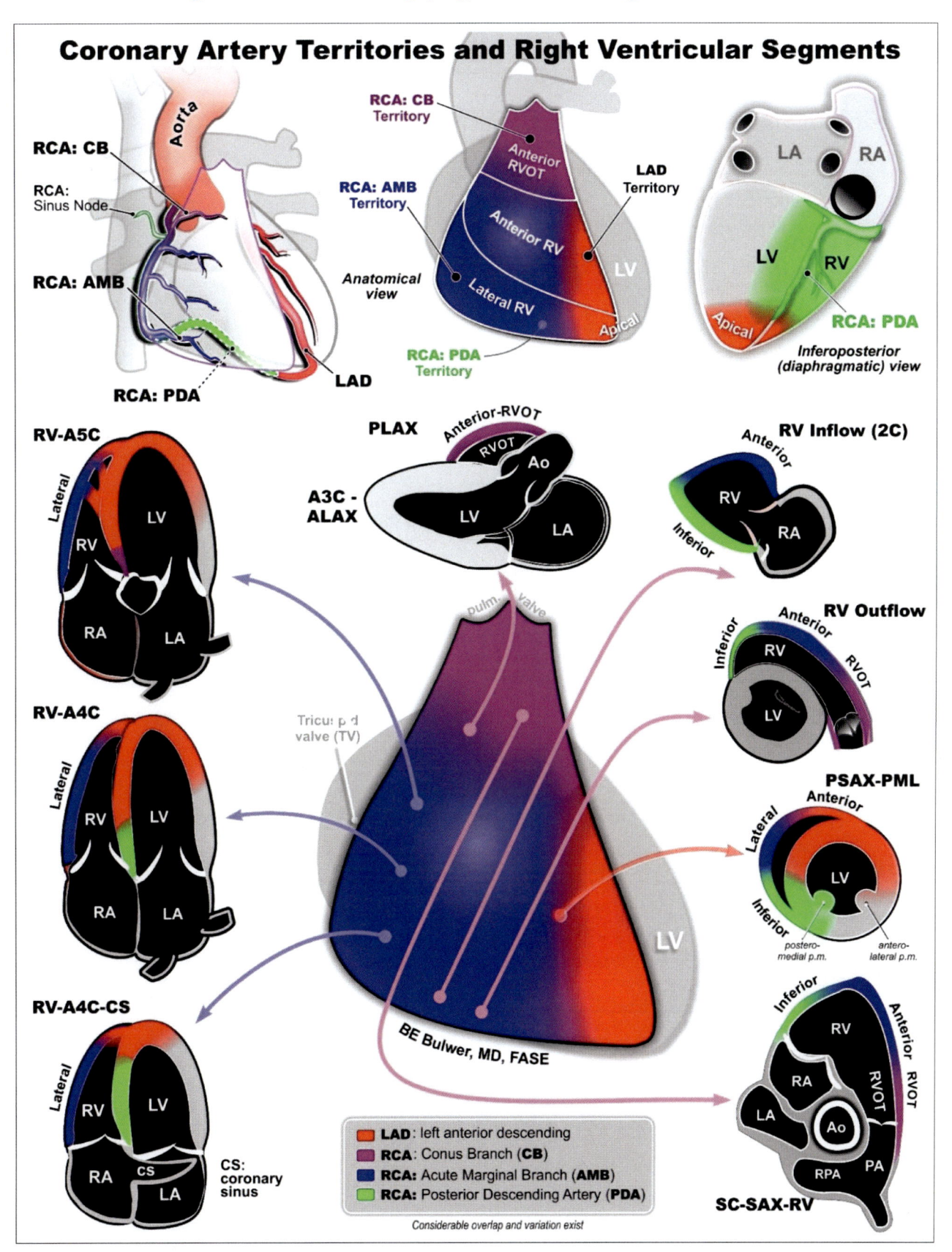

Fig. 75. Echocardiographic views of showing the major coronary artery supply to the right ventricular walls. Compare with Figs. 69-75.

Coronary Artery Assessment by Myocardial Contrast Echocardiography

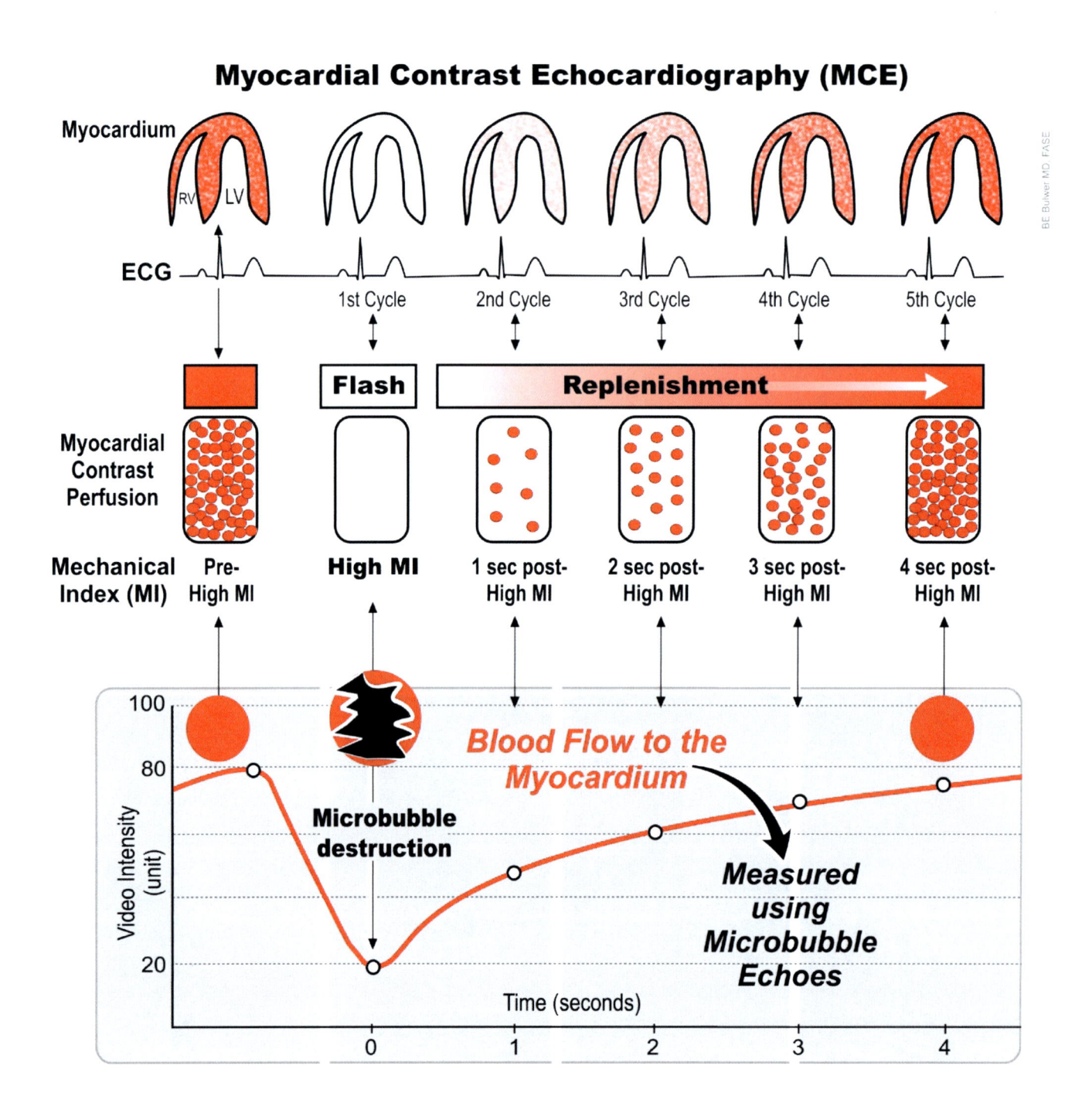

Ultrasound Contrast Agents: Basic Properties

Ultrasound Contrast Agents: Basic Properties

Ultrasound contrast agents are echo-enhancers engineered as a suspension of gas-filled microparticles (microbubbles), stabilized using an encapsulating shell of lipid, polymer, or protein.

Encapsulating Shell:
- Phospholipid, protein (albumin), polymer
- Surface properties: +/- biological or drug layer

Microbubbles
- **Microscopic**, strongly echogenic
- stable, reproducible contrast effect

Gas core: inert, low solubility gas
- Sulfur hexaflouride (Sonovue™)
- Perfluoropropane (Optison™)
- Octafluropropane (Definity™)
- Air (Levovist™, Cardiosphere™)

Chemical Formulae
- SF_6 (Sulfur hexaflouride)
- C_3F_8 (Octafluropropane)
- C_4F_{10} (Decafluorobutane)

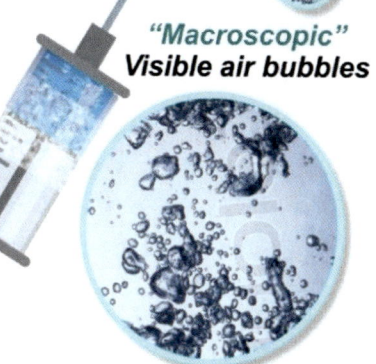

Microbubble diameter: 2-8 μm (micrometer)
Red blood cell (erythrocyte) diameter: 6-8 μm

"Macroscopic" Visible air bubbles

Agitated Saline
"Air Bubble Study"
- "Macrobubbles" Limited, very transient R-Heart contrast effct; cannot transit lungs, unless bypassed (R-L shunts)

Properties of The Ideal Ultrasound Contrast Agent

- **Strong Reflector:** Strongly echogenic to ultrasound when imaging using both the fundamental and harmonic frequencies.
- **Safe:** Established track record of safety
- **Ability to Pass Through the Lungs:** Small enough (like blood cells <8 μm) to flow unimpeded from the Pulmonary (Right-Heart), across the pulmonary microcirculation, into the Systemic (Left-Heart) circulation, the Left Ventricle (for LV Opacfication) and the Myocardium (heart muscle) for Myocardial Contrast Imaging.
- **Stability in Circulation:** Sufficiently stable following intravenous injection during its transit from the Pulmonary to Systemic circulation, and during ultrasonography Microbubble contrast agents have a natural propensity collapse or cavitate.
- **Stability during Exposure to Low Acoustic Power Ultrasound:** Mechanical effects of ultrasound (at normal acoustic power output) results in disruption and destruction of microbubbles. Hence, understanding the Mechanical Index is critical.
- **Size Uniformity, Homogenous and Reproducible Degree of Contrast:** Constrast microbubbles have a natural to collapse, shrink, and disappear.

BE Bulwer, MD, FASE

Fig. 76. Summary of the basic properties of ultrasound contrast agents that influence their role and utility in contrast-enhanced ultrasound. Assessment of regional wall motion abnormalities (RWMA) is an important component in the assessment of patients with coronary artery disease. Endocardial border definition using contrast agents, also called left ventricular opacification (LVO) to opacify the LV, is indicated when the endocardial border of two or more contiguous ventricular segments are not clearly seen. See Figs. 77-79.

Ultrasound Contrast Agents: Physical Principles

Ultrasound Contrast Agents: Physical Principles

- *Contrast Microbubbles are highly reflective suspensions injected intravenously to improve the diagnostic sensitivity of imaged structures by enhancing or creating a "contrast effect".*
- *Small enough (like blood cells <8 μm), remain intravascular, and excreted by the lungs.*

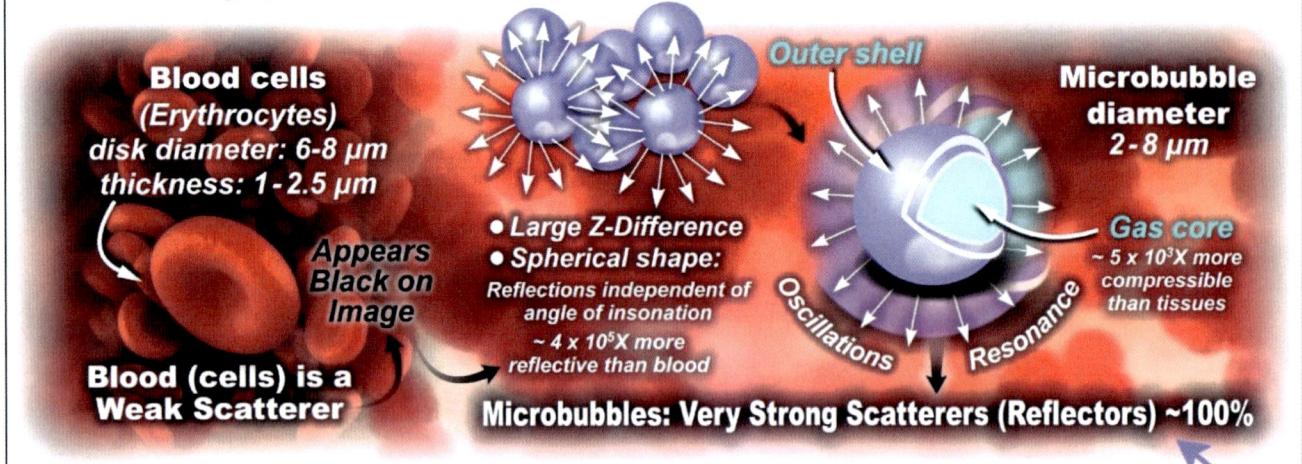

Blood cells (Erythrocytes) disk diameter: 6-8 μm; thickness: 1-2.5 μm. Appears Black on Image. **Blood (cells) is a Weak Scatterer**

- Large Z-Difference
- Spherical shape: Reflections independent of angle of insonation ~ 4×10^5X more reflective than blood

Outer shell — **Microbubble diameter 2-8 μm** — **Gas core** ~ 5×10^3X more compressible than tissues — Oscillations, Resonance

Microbubbles: Very Strong Scatterers (Reflectors) ~100%

Basis for the Contrast Effect of Microbubbles

Contrast Microbubbles are Very Strong Scatterers of Ultrasound

- **Strong reflections** (Rayleigh scattering) due to marked difference in Acoustic Impedance (Z) or mismatch between microbubbles and suspending medium (blood).
- **Gas Core:** This is the major determinant of microbubble reflectivity (echogenicity).

    Z(Gas) >>> Z(Blood) = Large Z-Difference = ~100% Reflection

- **Low Solubility Gases:** Slows the diffusion of gas, which lengthens the duration of contrast (low Ostwald coefficient of gas solubility).
- **Encapsulating Shell:** Outer shell slows diffusion of gases, which lengthens the duration of contrast (Epstein-Plesset model for gas microparticle dissolution). Spherical shape ensures scattering regardless of insonation angle.
- **Linear vs. Non-Linear Behavior:** Microbubbles are <u>highly compressible</u> due to their gas content. <u>At LOW acoustic pressures</u>, they contract and expand (volumetric oscillation), exhibiting linear behavior or stable cavitation.
  <u>At progressively HIGHER acoustic pressures</u>, microbubbles bulge or expand more than they contract (oscillate assymetrically), exhibit non-linear behavior, generate harmonic frequencies, progressing to abrupt bubble destruction (inertial cavitation).
- **Stronger Harmonics:** Microbubbles generate stronger harmonics than tissues, i.e. Contrast Microbubble Harmonics >>> Tissue Harmonics. This is the basis for
  Contrast Harmonic Imaging. <u>This also occurs at lower acoustic pressures</u>, e.g. at Mechanical Index (MI) < 0.3 (compare tissue harmonics, which arise only at higher MI).
- Images created from Contrast Microbubble Harmonics: **Contrast Harmonic Imaging**, provide greater image contrast (with adjacent tissues)

BE Bulwer, MD, FASE

Fig. 77. Summary of the physical properties of contrast agents and their impact in contrast-enhanced ultrasound. Contrast agents are also used to directly assess myocardial blood flow using myocardial contrast echocardiography (MCE), also called myocardial perfusion imaging. See Fig. 80

Clinical Utility of Contrast Agents in Echocardiography I

Agitated Saline "Bubble Study"

R-Heart Opacification

- Rapid injection of a bolus of agitated saline - air contrast "macrobubbles" that transiently fill the R-Heart Chambers.
- Air Bubbles are too large to traverse the lung (pulmonary microcirculation), hence restricted to the R-Heart chambers.

MI 0.8 - 1.4
Normal B-Mode

R-L shunts
"Hole in the Heart"
PFO, ASD*
Pulmonary AVM**

Air Bubbles appearing in L-Heart Chambers indicates Abnormal R to L shunt

Air Bubbles — Right (R) Lung — Left (L) Lung

* Patent Foramen Ovale,
* Atrial Septal Defect
** Arteriovenous Malformation

Left Ventricular Opacification: Endocardial Border Definition

Endocardial border Not Easily Defined

MI 0.8 - 1.4
Normal B-Mode

For more accurate assessment of left ventricular (LV) volumes

LV Opacification with Contrast Microbubbles

Low MI < 0.3 → More Accurate Assessment

Endocardial border Better Definition — Myocardium

Myocardial Perfusion Imaging with Contrast Ultrasound
To assess blood flow (perfusion) to the myocardium

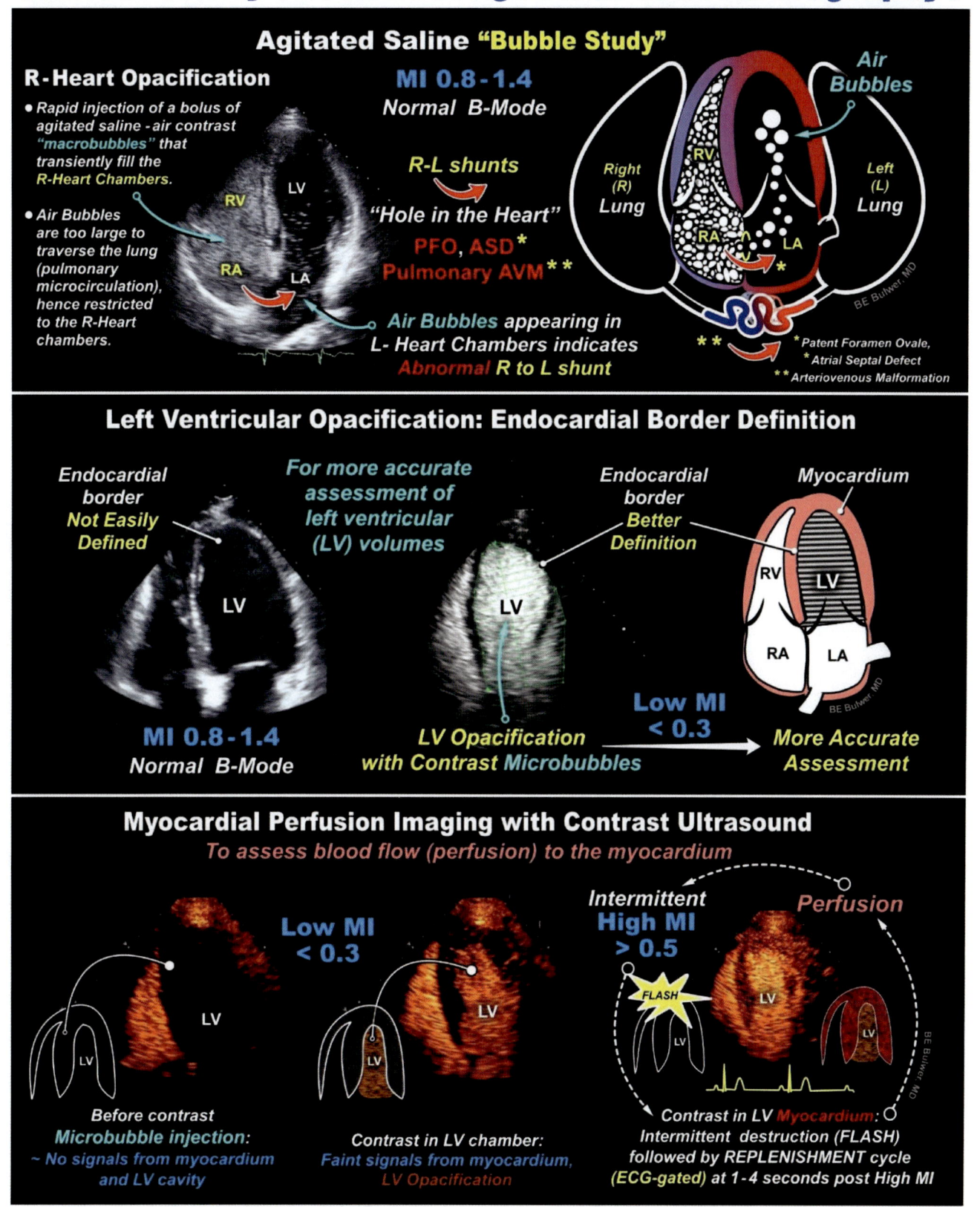

Before contrast Microbubble injection:
~ No signals from myocardium and LV cavity

Low MI < 0.3
Contrast in LV chamber:
Faint signals from myocardium, LV Opacification

Intermittent High MI > 0.5
Perfusion
FLASH

Contrast in LV Myocardium: Intermittent destruction (FLASH) followed by REPLENISHMENT cycle (ECG-gated) at 1-4 seconds post High MI

Fig. 78. Three different applications of contrast agents in echocardiography: *Above,* Right ventricular (RV) opacification using agitated saline contrast for evaluation of right-to-left shuts; *Middle,* Left ventricular (LV) opacification for endocardial border definition and evaluation of masses in the LV chamber, *Below,* Myocardial perfusion imaging for evaluation of blood flow to the heart in coronary artery disease.

Contrast Echocardiography: Optimizing Image Acquisition

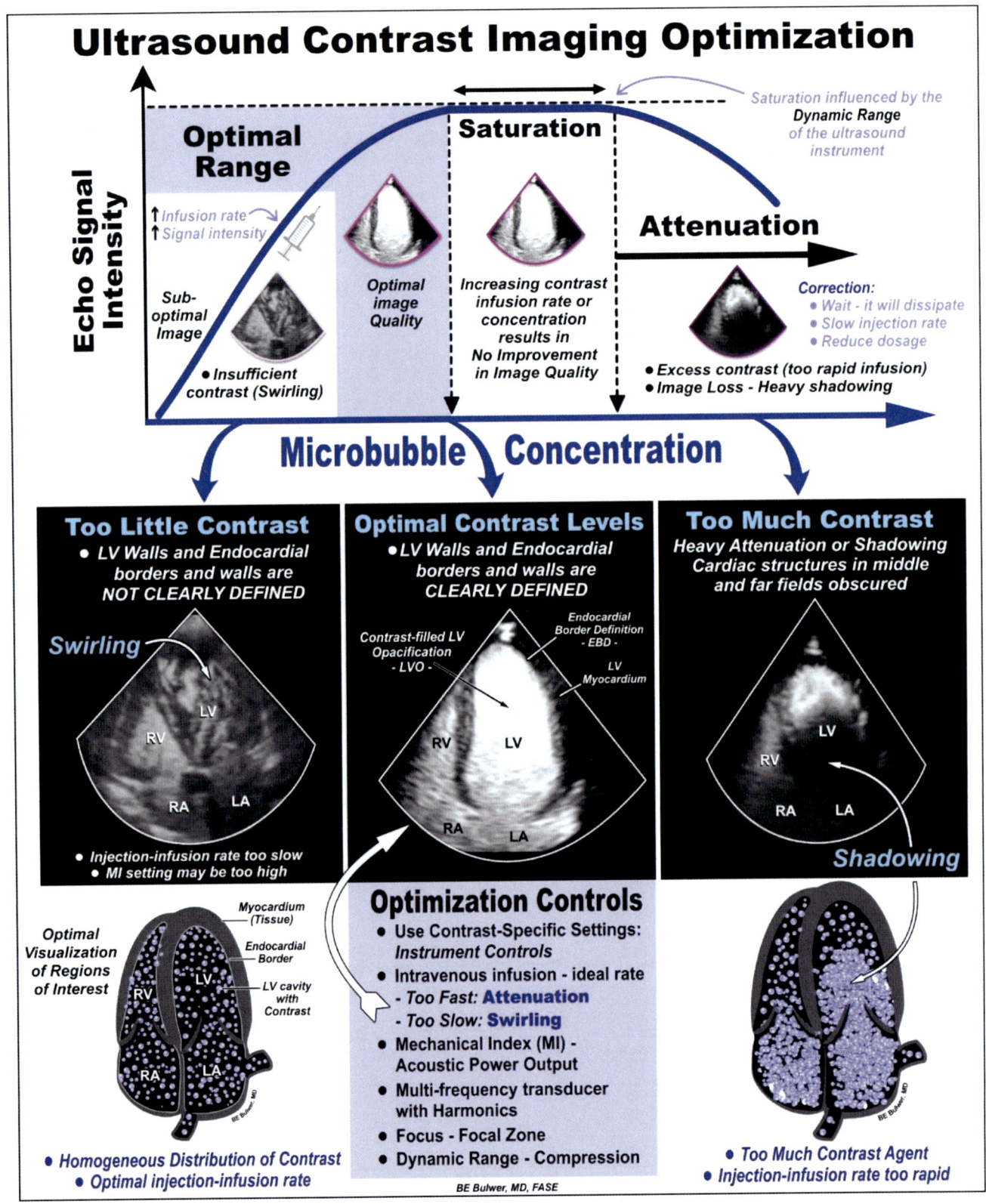

Fig. 79. **Contrast-enhanced echocardiography:** Image optimization protocols, controls, and caveats. Regional wall motion assessment (RWMA) is important in the echocardiographic assessment of coronary artery disease. Visualization of the endocardial border is critical in this assessment. Therefore, left ventricular opacification (LVO) using contrast agents is performed when visualization of the LV segments is suboptimal. Contrast agents are now routinely employed during stress echocardiography for assessment of RWMA (Figs. 32-34, Table 1).

Myocardial Blood Flow using Contrast Ultrasound

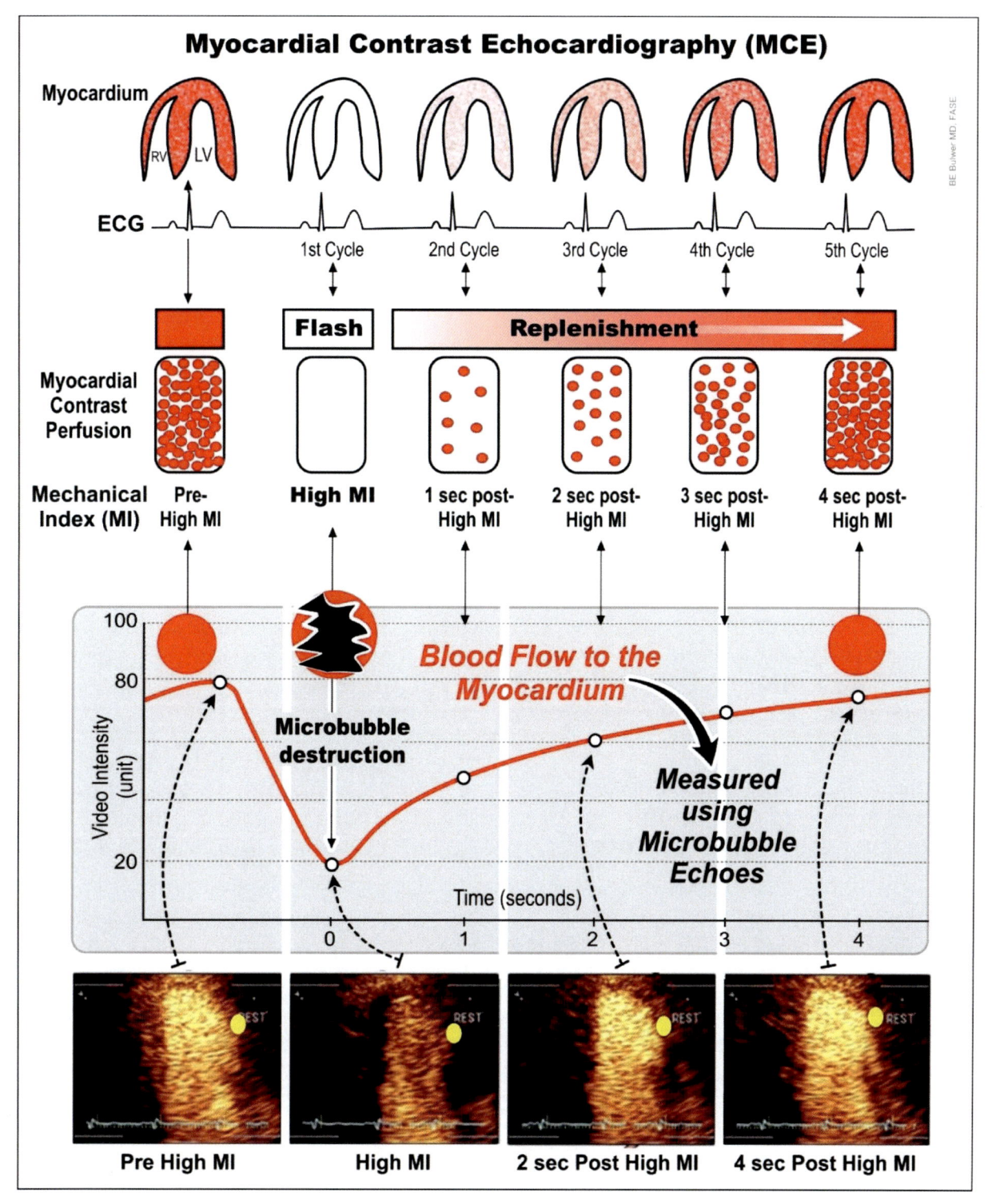

Fig. 80. Myocardial Contrast Echocardiography (MCE)—Myocardial Perfusion Imaging: Blood flow to the myocardium (perfusion) can be non-invasively assessed in real-time using a high–mechanical index (MI) technique. *From left to right columns:* Following injection of microbubble contrast agent **(Pre-High MI)** note normal perfusion to the myocardium. During the **High MI "flash"**, microbubbles are completely destroyed. Normal replenishment of contrast agent, representing blood flow, normally occurs within 4 seconds following the high MI flash. This serves as the basis for measuring perfusion to the heart, hence its utility in the evaluation of coronary artery disease. Quantification algorithms and image subtraction techniques can provide accurate estimates of myocardial perfusion, e.g. **slope times peak** or **peak plateau myocardial contrast intensity**.

References

1. Altiok E, Tiemann S, Becker M, et al. *Myocardial deformation imaging by two-dimensional speckle-tracking echocardiography for prediction of global and segmental functional changes after acute myocardial infarction: a comparison with late gadolinium enhancement cardiac magnetic resonance.* J Am Soc Echocardiogr. 2014;27:249-257.

2. Biering-Sørensen T, Hoffmann S, Mogelvang R, et al. *Myocardial strain analysis by 2-dimensional speckle tracking echocardiography improves diagnostics of coronary artery stenosis in stable angina pectoris.* Circ Cardiovasc Imaging. 2014;7:58–65.

3. Bulwer BE. *Transthoracic Echocardiography: Foundations of Image Acquisition and Interpretation.* Echo Stethoscope Academy. Boston, MA. 2020.

4. Cerqueira MD, Weissman NJ, Dilsizian V, et al. *Standardized Myocardial Segmentation and Nomenclature.* Circulation. 2002;105:539–542.

5. Cortigiani L, Urluescu ML, Coltelli M, Carpeggiani C, Bovenzi F, Picano E. *Apparent Declining Prognostic Value of a Negative Stress Echocardiography Based on Regional Wall Motion Abnormalities in Patients With Normal Resting Left Ventricular Function Due to the Changing Referral Profile of the Population Under Study.* Circ Cardiovasc Imaging. 2019;12(6):e008564.

6. Edvardsen T, Helle-Valle T, Smiseth OA. Systolic dysfunction in heart failure with normal ejection fraction: speckle-tracking echocardiography. Prog Cardiovasc Dis. 2006;49(3):207-214.

7. Gulel O, Akcay M, Soylu K, et al. *Left Ventricular Myocardial Deformation Parameters Are Affected by Coronary Slow Flow Phenomenon: A Study of Speckle Tracking Echocardiography.* Echocardiography. 2016;33:714-723.

8. Hoffmann U, Ferencik M, Udelson JE, et al. *Prognostic Value of Noninvasive Cardiovascular Testing in Patients with Stable Chest Pain: Insights from the PROMISE Trial (Prospective Multicenter Imaging Study for Evaluation of Chest Pain).* Circulation. 2017;135:2320-2332.

9. Hunziker PR, Picard MH, Jander N, Scherrer-Crosbie M, Pfisterer M, Buser PT. *Regional wall motion assessment in stress echocardiography by tissue Doppler bull's-eyes.* J Am Soc Echocardiogr. 1999;12(3):196-202.

10. Kurt M, Tanboga IH, Aksakal E. *Two-Dimensional Strain Imaging: Basic principles and Technical Consideration.* Eurasian J Med. 2014;46:126-130.

11. Lancellotti P, Pellikka PA, Budts W, et al. *The Clinical Use of Stress Echocardiography in Non-Ischaemic Heart Disease: Recommendations from the European Association of Cardiovascular Imaging and the American Society of Echocardiography.* J Am Soc Echocardiogr. 2017;30:101-138.

12. Lang RM, Badano LP, Tsang W, Adams DH, Agricola E, Buck T, Faletra FF, Franke A, Hung J, de Isla LP, Kamp O, Kasprzak JD, Lancellotti P, Marwick TH, McCulloch ML, Monaghan MJ, Nihoyannopoulos P, Pandian NG, Pellikka PA, Pepi M, Roberson DA,

Shernan SK, Shirali GS, Sugeng L, Ten Cate FJ, Van-nan MA, Zamorano JL, Zoghbi WA; American Society of Echocardiography; European Association of Echocardiography. *EAE/ASE recommendations for image acquisition and display using three-dimensional echocardiography*. J Am Soc Echocardiogr. 2012;25:3-46.

13. Lang RM, Badano LP, Mor-Avi V, et al. *Recommendations for cardiac chamber quantification by echocardiography in adults: an update from the American Society of Echocardiography and the European Association of Cardiovascular Imaging*. J Am Soc Echocardiogr. 2015;28:1-39.

14. Mada RO, Duchenne J, Voigt JU. *Tissue Doppler, strain and strain rate in ischemic heart disease "how I do it"*. Cardiovasc Ultrasound. 2014;12:38. Published 2014 Sep 18. doi:10.1186/1476-7120-12-38.

15. Park JH. *Two-dimensional Echocardiographic Assessment of Myocardial Strain: Important Echocardiographic Parameter Readily Useful in Clinical Field*. Korean Circ J. 2019 Oct;49(10):908-931.

16. Pellikka PA, Nagueh SF, Elhendy AA, Kuehl CA, Sawada SG; American Society of Echocardiography. *American Society of Echocardiography recommendations for performance, interpretation, and application of stress echocardiography*. J Am Soc Echocardiogr. 2007, 20:1021-41.

17. Picano E, Ciampi Q, Wierzbowska-Drabik K, Urluescu ML, Morrone D, Carpeggiani C. *The new clinical standard of integrated quadruple stress echocardiography with ABCD protocol*. Cardiovasc Ultrasound. 2018;16(1):22.

18. Picano E. *Stress echocardiography*. 5th ed. Springer, Berlin, 2009:31-42.

19. Sicari R, Cortigiani L. *The clinical use of stress echocardiography in ischemic heart disease. Cardiovasc Ultrasound*. 2017;15(1):7.

20. Takeuchi M, Nakazono A. *Coronary Artery Imaging with Transthoracic Doppler Echocardiography*. Curr Cardiol Rep. 2016;18(7):63.

21. Feigenbaum H, Armstrong WF, Ryan T. *Contrast Echocardiography.* In: Armstrong WF, Ryan T, ed. Feigenbaum's Echocardiography. 8th ed. Baltimore: Wolters Kluwer- Lippincott Williams & Wilkins, 2019:38–60.

22. Karogiannis N, Senior R. *Contrast echocardiography for detection of myocardial perfusion abnormalities: A clinical perspective*. Herz. 2017; 42:287-294.

23. Lang RM, Badano LP, Tsang W, et al. *EAE/ASE recommendations for image acquisition and display using three-dimensional echocardiography*. Euro Heart J of Cardiovasc Imaging; 2012,13:1–46.

24. Lindner JR. *A Practical Approach to Contrast Echocardiography*. Expert Analysis: Latest in Cardiology. American College of Cardiology. July 10, 2017.

25. Lindner JR. *Contrast Echocardiography: The Bubbles and How We Image Them*. American Society of Echocardiography. YouTube-ASE 360. April 12, 2016.

26. Lindner JR. *Physical Properties of Microbubble Ultrasound Contrast Agents.* In: Lang RM, Goldstein SA, Kronzon I, Khanderia BK, Mor-Avi V. ASE's Comprehensive Echocardiography. Philadelphia, Elsevier. 2016:94-97.

27. Marwick TH, Taylor AJ. *Contrast-Specific Imaging Without Contrast: An Echocardiographic Technique for the Detection of Myocardial Scar*. JACC Cardiovasc Imaging. 2016 Nov; 9:1252-1254.

Glossary: Abbreviations and Symbols

D; 1-D	one-dimensional (M-mode)
2D; 2-D	two-dimensional
3D; 3-D	three-dimensional
4C	four-chamber
A-long	apical long-axis
A2C	apical two-chamber
A3C	apical three-chamber
A4C	apical four-chamber
A5C	apical five-chamber
AC	aortic closure
AF	atrial fibrillation
AHA	American Heart Association
ALAX	apical long-axis view (or A3C)
AML	anterior mitral valve leaflet
Ao	aortic or aorta
AR	aortic regurgitation
AS	aortic stenosis
ASE	American Society of Echocardiography
ATVL	anterior tricuspid valve leaflet
AV	atrioventricular
CAD	coronary artery disease
CFD	color flow Doppler
CMR	cardiac magnetic resonance imaging
CS	coronary sinus
CW	continuous-wave
DA	descending aorta
echo	echocardiography
endo	endocardium
Hv	hepatic vein
IAS	interatrial septum
IV	intravenous
IVC	inferior vena cava
IVCCI	inferior vena cava collapsibility index
IVCT	isovolumic contraction time
IVRT	isovolumic relaxation time
IVS	interventricular septum
LA	left atrium
LAA	left atrial appendage
LAD	left anterior descending coronary artery
LAO	left anterior oblique
LCC	left coronary cusp
LCx	left circumflex coronary artery
LLPV	left lower pulmonary vein
LMCA	left main coronary artery
LPA	left pulmonary artery
LSPV	left superior pulmonary vein
LUPV	left upper pulmonary vein
LV	left ventricle
LVEDP	left ventricular end-diastolic pressure
LVEF	left ventricular ejection fraction
LVH	left ventricular hypertrophy
LVID	left ventricular internal dimension
LVOT	left ventricular outflow tract
M-mode	motion-mode (depth versus time)
MAC	mitral annular calcification
MI	myocardial infarction
MO	mitral opening
MR	mitral regurgitation
MS	mitral stenosis
MV	mitral valve
MVA	mitral valve area
MVL	mitral valve leaflet
MVR	mitral valve replacement
NCC	noncoronary cusp
PA	pulmonary artery
PAB	pulmonary artery bifurcation
PAP	pulmonary artery pressure
PDA	patent ductus arteriosus or posterior descending artery
PLAX	parasternal long-axis
PLSVC	persistent left superior vena cava
PM	papillary muscle
PMVL	posterior mitral valve leaflet
PR	pulmonary regurgitation
PS	pulmonary stenosis
PSAX	parasternal short-axis
PV	pulmonary valve
Pv	pulmonary vein
PW	pulsed-wave
PWT	posterior wall thickness
RA	right atrium
RAO	right anterior oblique
RCA	right coronary artery
RCC	right coronary cusp
RLPV	right lower pulmonary vein
RPA	right pulmonary artery
RSPV	right superior pulmonary vein
RSV	regurgitant stroke volume
RUPV	right upper pulmonary vein
RV	right ventricle
RVOT	right ventricular outflow tract
SAX	short-axis
SC	subcostal
SC-4C	subcostal four-chamber
SC-LAX	subcostal long-axis
SC-SAX	subcostal short-axis
SSN	suprasternal notch
ST	septal thickness
SVC	superior vena cava
TR	tricuspid regurgitation
TS	tricuspid stenosis
TTE	transthoracic echocardiography
TV	tricuspid valve

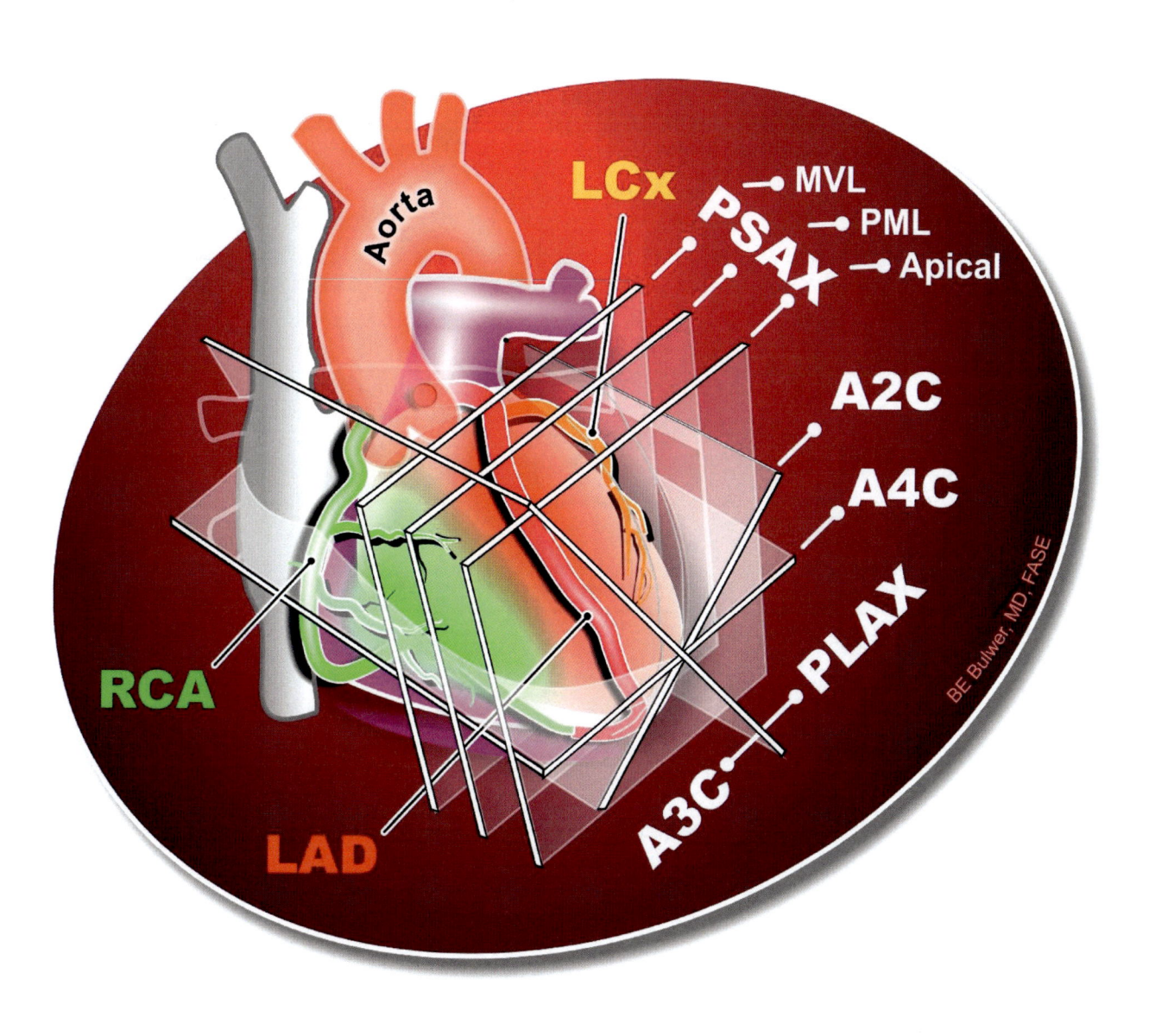

Coronary Artery Territories

Polar "Bull's Eye" Plot of the Left Ventricular (LV) Myocardial Wall Segments

LV Segments	Total Number of Segments	Numbers
Basal LV Segments	6	1-6
Mid LV Segments	6	7-12
Apical Segments	4	13-16
Apical Cap	1	17
Total	N = 17	1-17

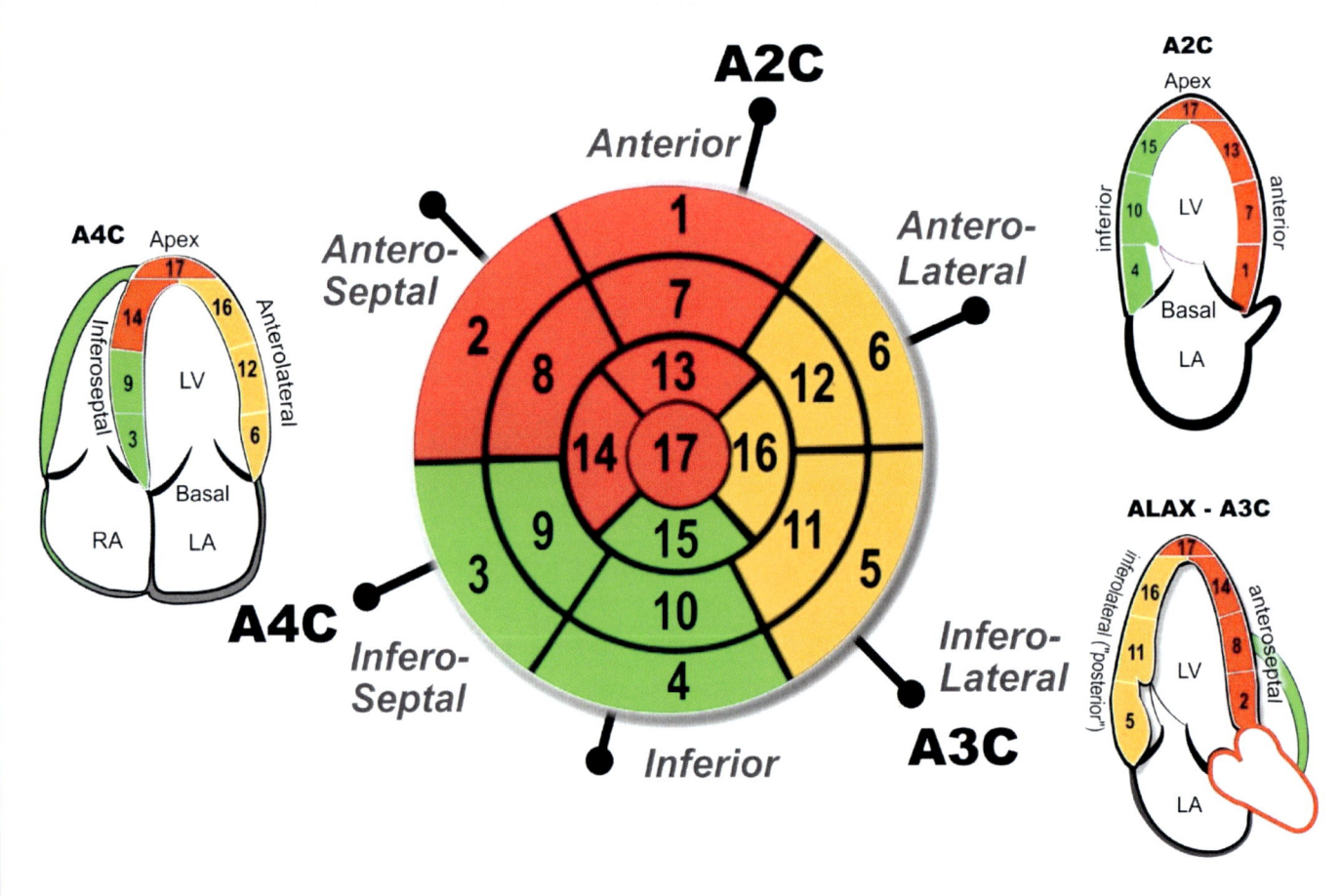

Basal
1. basal anterior
2. basal anteroseptal
3. basal inferoseptal
4. basal inferior
5. basal inferolateral
6. basal anterolateral

Mid-LV
7. mid anterior
8. mid anteroseptal
9. mid inferoseptal
10. mid inferior
11. mid inferolateral
12. mid anterolatral

Apical
13. apical anterior
14. apical septal
15. apical inferior
16. apical lateral

Apex
17. apex

BE Bulwer, MD, FASE

Left Ventricular (LV) Segments

LAD, left anterior descending coronary artery; **RCA/PDA**, right coronary and posteior descending artery; **LCA**, left circumflex artery

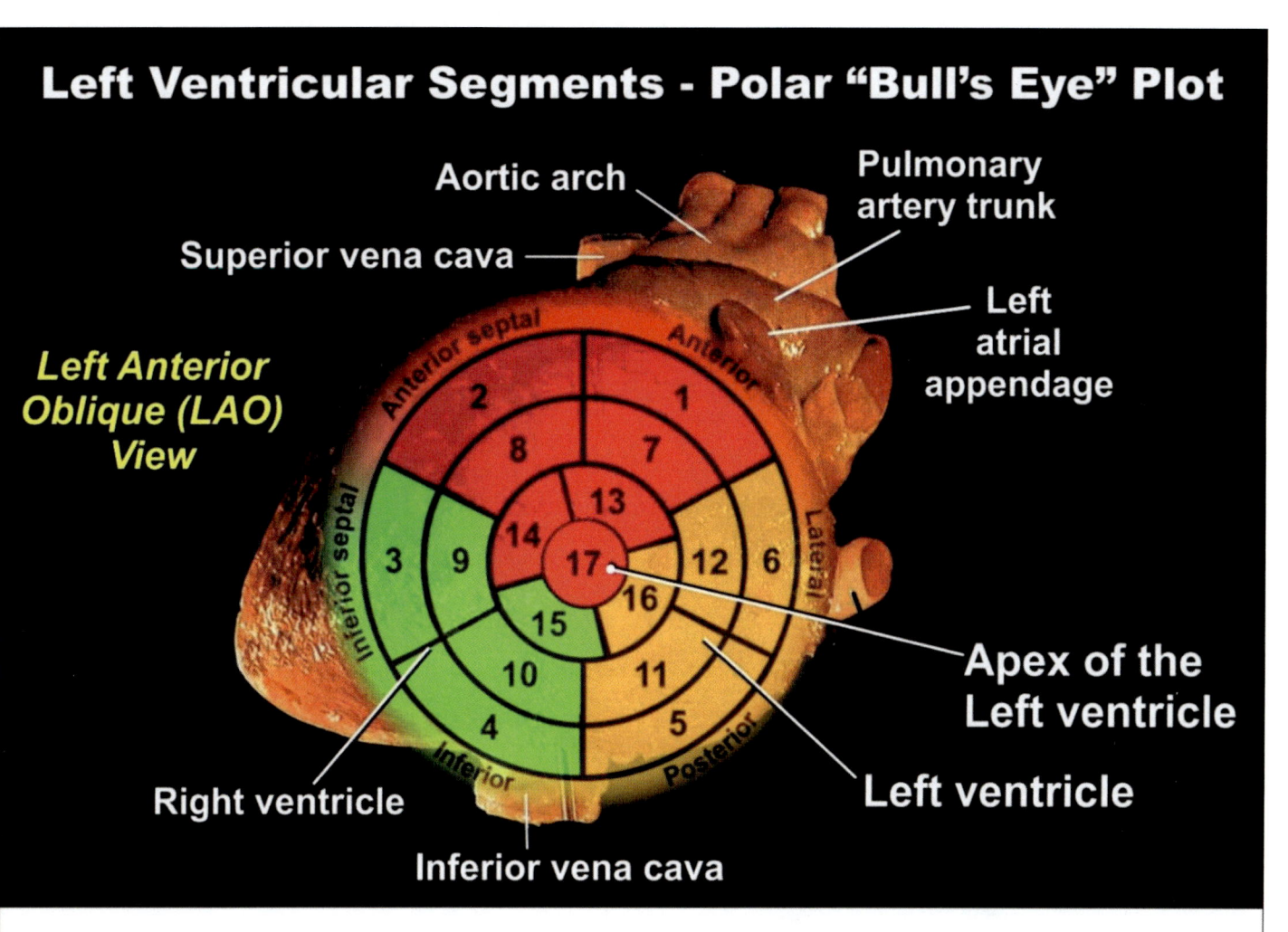

Coronary Artery Territories

Left Ventricular Segments – Polar "Bull's Eye" Plot

Left Anterior Oblique (LAO) View

- Aortic arch
- Pulmonary artery trunk
- Superior vena cava
- Left atrial appendage
- Apex of the Left ventricle
- Left ventricle
- Right ventricle
- Inferior vena cava

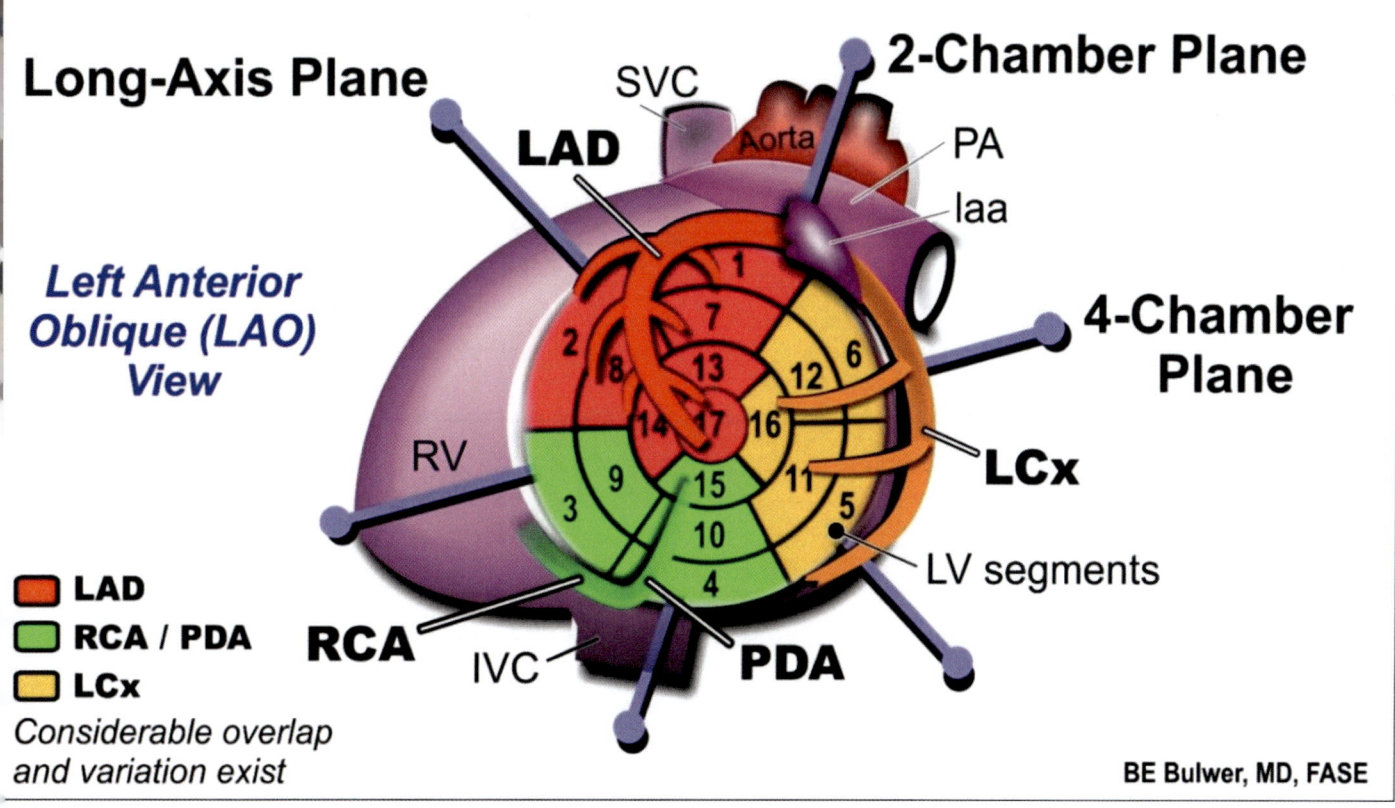

Long-Axis Plane · 2-Chamber Plane · 4-Chamber Plane

Left Anterior Oblique (LAO) View

- SVC
- LAD
- Aorta
- PA
- laa
- RV
- LCx
- RCA
- IVC
- PDA
- LV segments

- 🟥 LAD
- 🟩 RCA / PDA
- 🟨 LCx

Considerable overlap and variation exist

BE Bulwer, MD, FASE

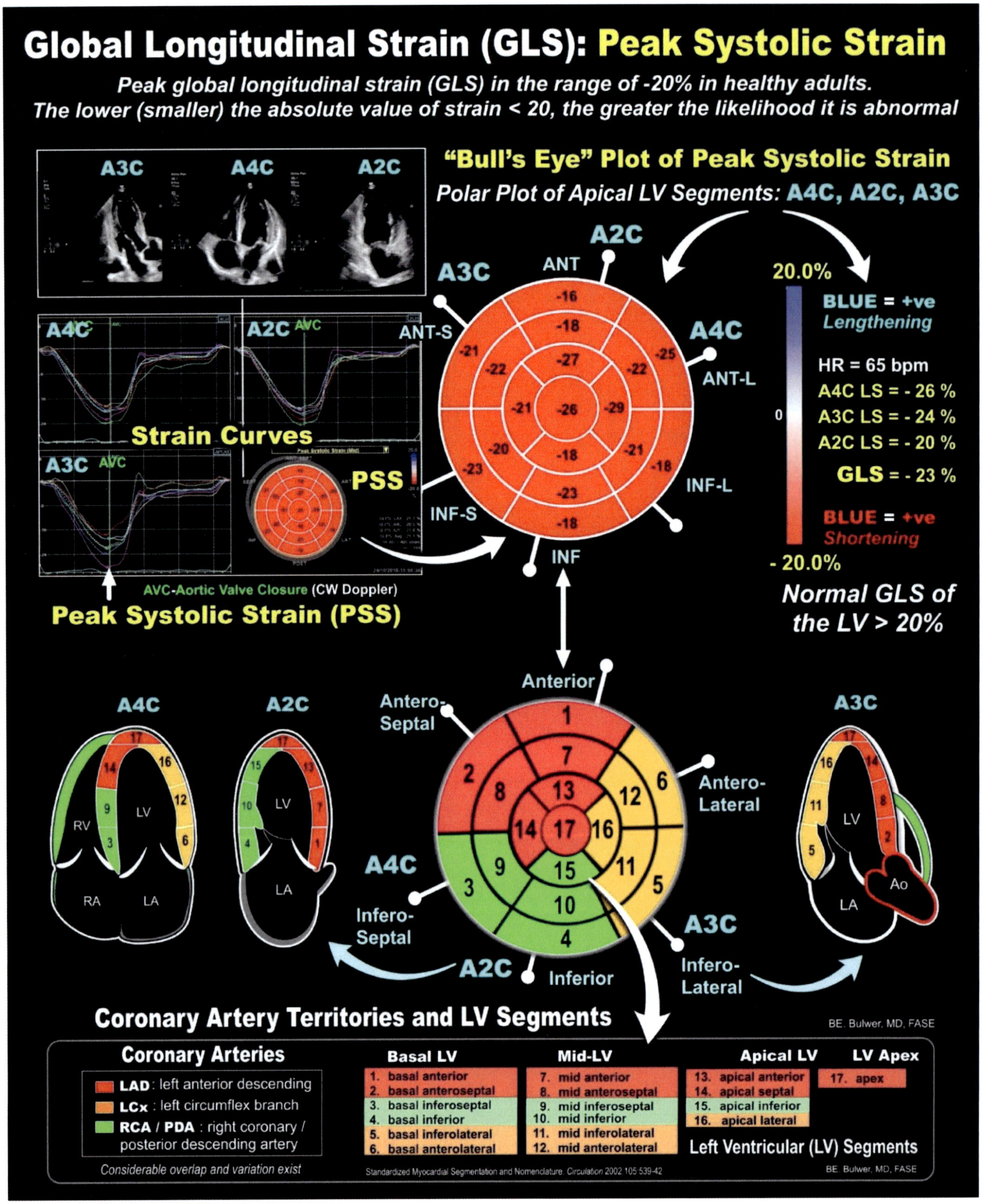
Global Longitudinal Strain (GLS): Peak Systolic Strain
Peak global longitudinal strain (GLS) in the range of -20% in healthy adults.
The lower (smaller) the absolute value of strain < 20, the greater the likelihood it is abnormal
A3C
A4C
A2C
A4C
A2C AVC
A3C AVC
Strain Curves
PSS
AVC-Aortic Valve Closure (CW Doppler)
Peak Systolic Strain (PSS)
"Bull's Eye" Plot of Peak Systolic Strain
Polar Plot of Apical LV Segments: A4C, A2C, A3C
A2C
A3C
ANT
ANT-S
A4C
ANT-L
INF-S
INF-L
INF
-16
-18
-21
-22
-27
-22
-25
-21
-26
-29
-20
-18
-21
-23
-23
-18
-18
20.0%
BLUE = +ve
Lengthening
0
HR = 65 bpm
A4C LS = - 26 %
A3C LS = - 24 %
A2C LS = - 20 %
GLS = - 23 %
BLUE = +ve
Shortening
- 20.0%
Normal GLS of the LV > 20%
A4C
A2C
A3C
RV
LV
RA
LA
LV
LA
LV
LA
Ao
Anterior
Antero-Septal
Antero-Lateral
A4C
Infero-Septal
A2C
Inferior
A3C
Infero-Lateral
Coronary Artery Territories and LV Segments
BE. Bulwer, MD, FASE
Coronary Arteries
LAD: left anterior descending
LCx: left circumflex branch
RCA / PDA: right coronary / posterior descending artery
Considerable overlap and variation exist
Basal LV
1. basal anterior
2. basal anteroseptal
3. basal inferoseptal
4. basal inferior
5. basal inferolateral
6. basal anterolateral
Mid-LV
7. mid anterior
8. mid anteroseptal
9. mid inferoseptal
10. mid inferior
11. mid inferolateral
12. mid anterolateral
Apical LV
13. apical anterior
14. apical septal
15. apical inferior
16. apical lateral
LV Apex
17. apex
Left Ventricular (LV) Segments
Standardized Myocardial Segmentation and Nomenclature. Circulation 2002 105:539-42
BE. Bulwer, MD, FASE

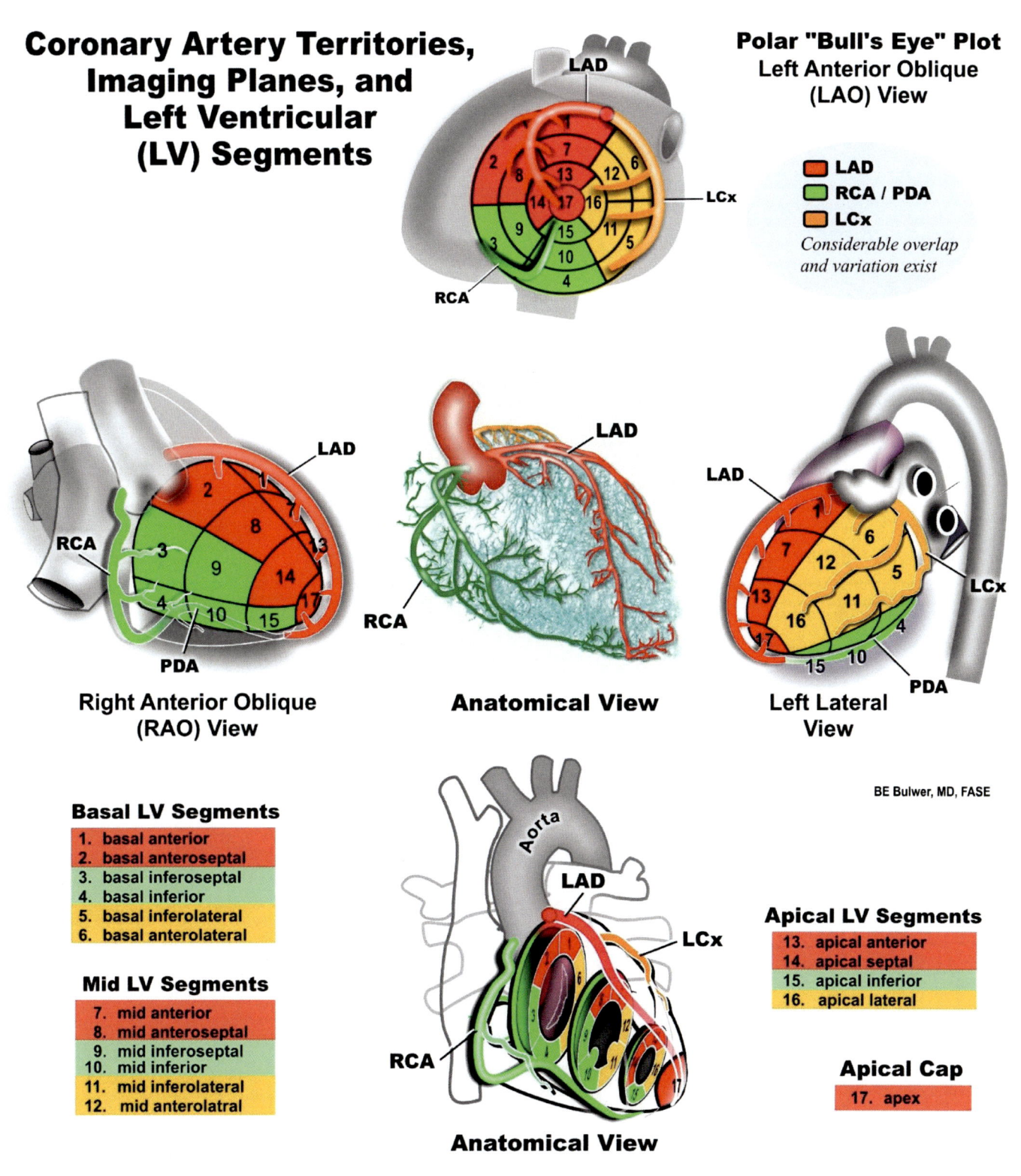

Coronary Artery Territories, Imaging Planes, and Left Ventricular (LV) Segments

Polar "Bull's Eye" Plot
Left Anterior Oblique (LAO) View

- LAD
- RCA / PDA
- LCx

Considerable overlap and variation exist

Right Anterior Oblique (RAO) View

Anatomical View

Left Lateral View

BE Bulwer, MD, FASE

Basal LV Segments
1. basal anterior
2. basal anteroseptal
3. basal inferoseptal
4. basal inferior
5. basal inferolateral
6. basal anterolateral

Mid LV Segments
7. mid anterior
8. mid anteroseptal
9. mid inferoseptal
10. mid inferior
11. mid inferolateral
12. mid anterolatral

Anatomical View

Apical LV Segments
13. apical anterior
14. apical septal
15. apical inferior
16. apical lateral

Apical Cap
17. apex

LAD, left anterior descending coronary artery; **RCA/PDA**, right coronary and posteior descending artery; **LCA**, left circumflex artery

Wall Motion Assessment: RCA Territory

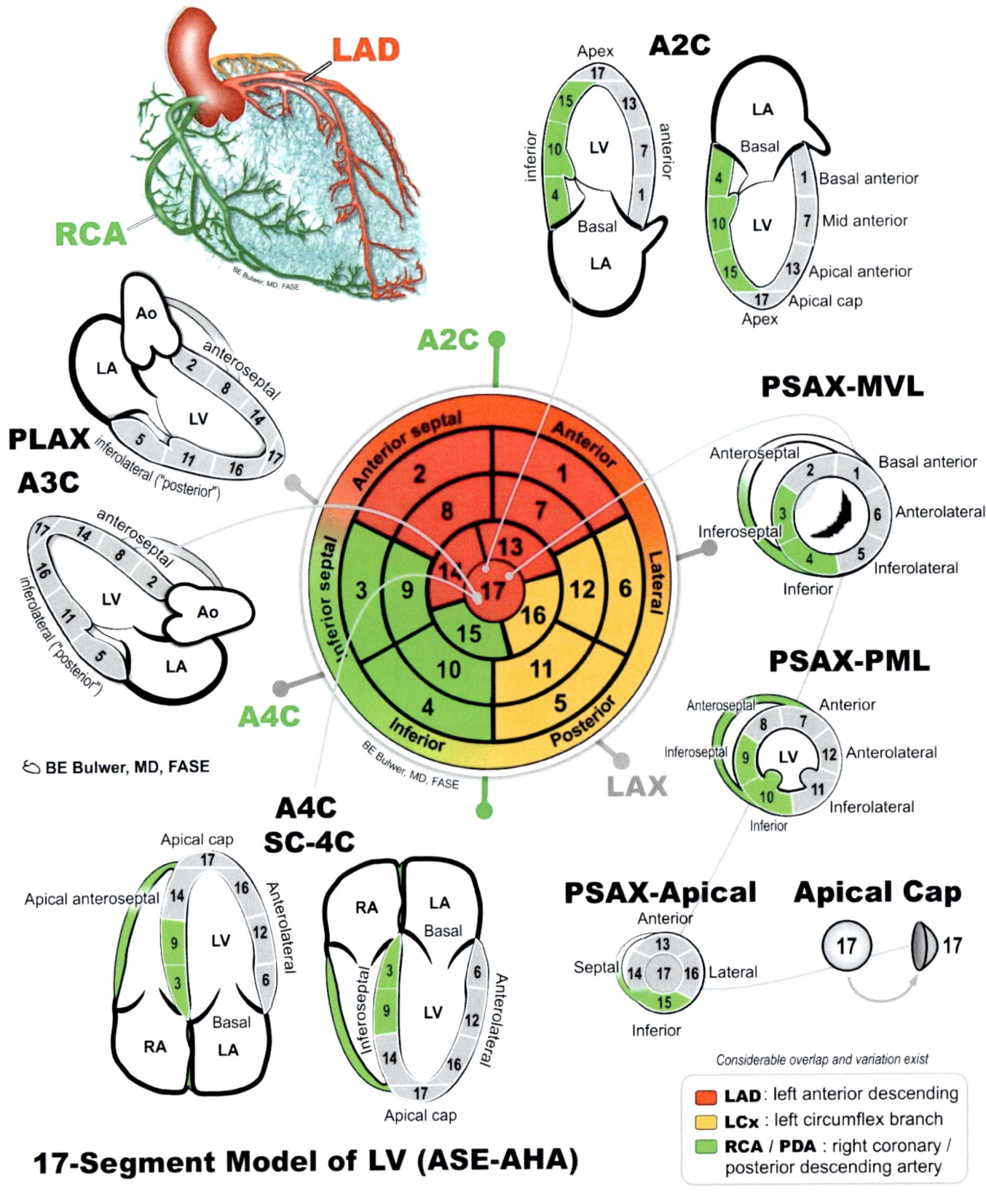

17-Segment Model of LV (ASE-AHA)

Considerable overlap and variation exist

- **LAD**: left anterior descending
- **LCx**: left circumflex branch
- **RCA / PDA**: right coronary / posterior descending artery

BE Bulwer, MD, FASE

Coronary Artery Territories

Wall Motion Assessment: LCx Territory

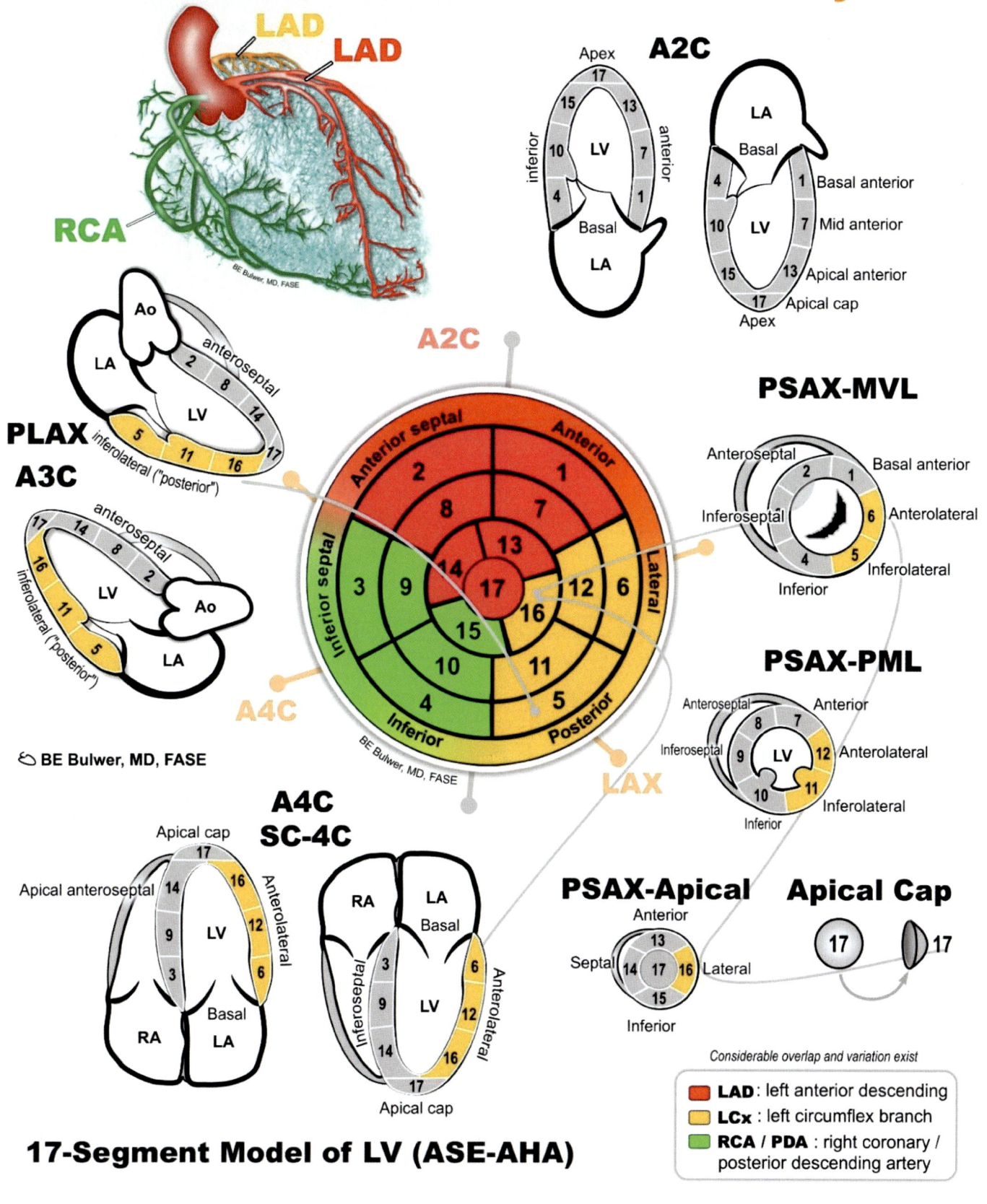

17-Segment Model of LV (ASE-AHA)

Considerable overlap and variation exist

- **LAD**: left anterior descending
- **LCx**: left circumflex branch
- **RCA / PDA**: right coronary / posterior descending artery

© BE Bulwer, MD, FASE

97

98 Echocardiography Illustrated

Wall Motion Assessment: LAD Territory

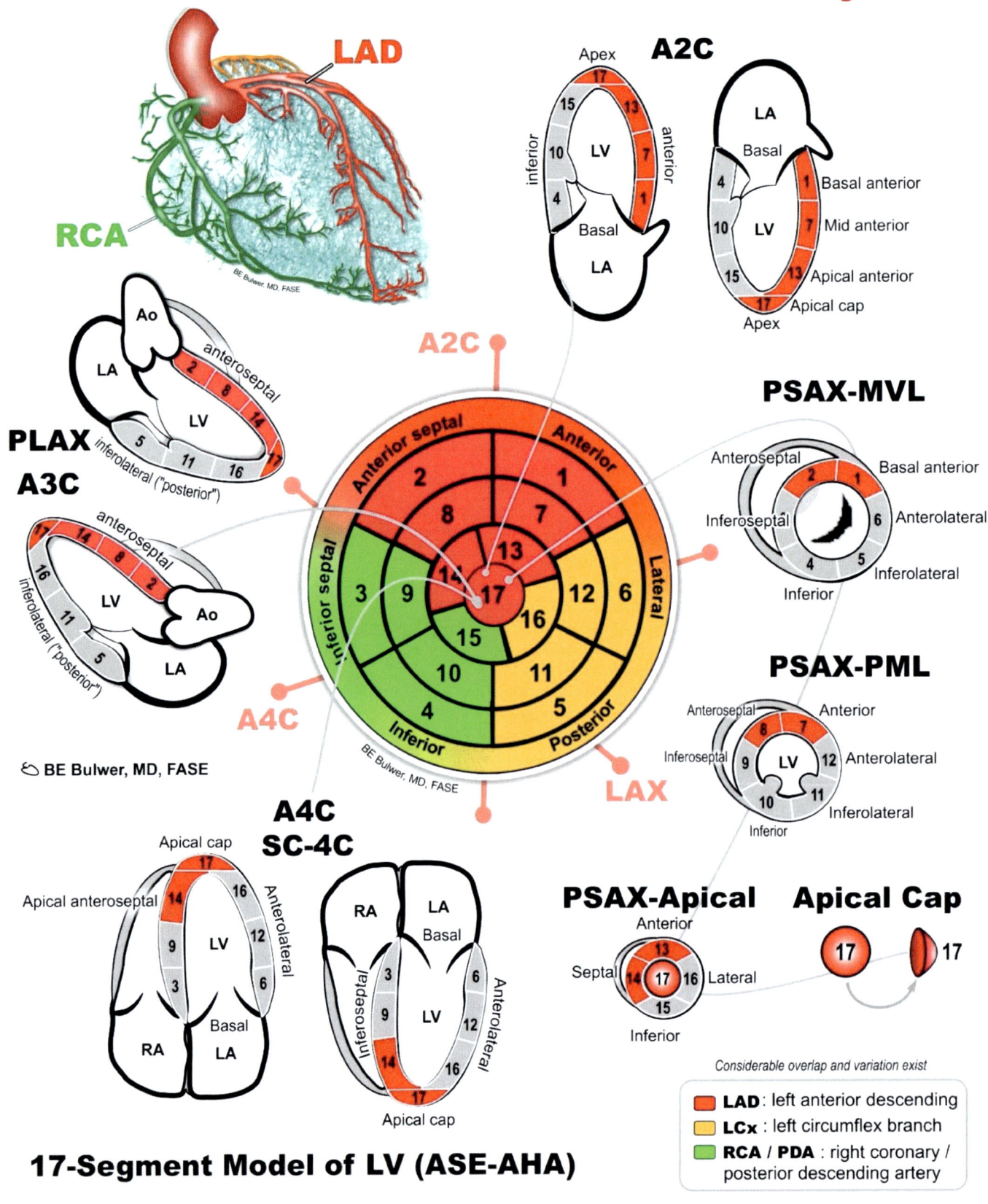

17-Segment Model of LV (ASE-AHA)

BE Bulwer, MD, FASE

Considerable overlap and variation exist

- **LAD**: left anterior descending
- **LCx**: left circumflex branch
- **RCA / PDA**: right coronary / posterior descending artery

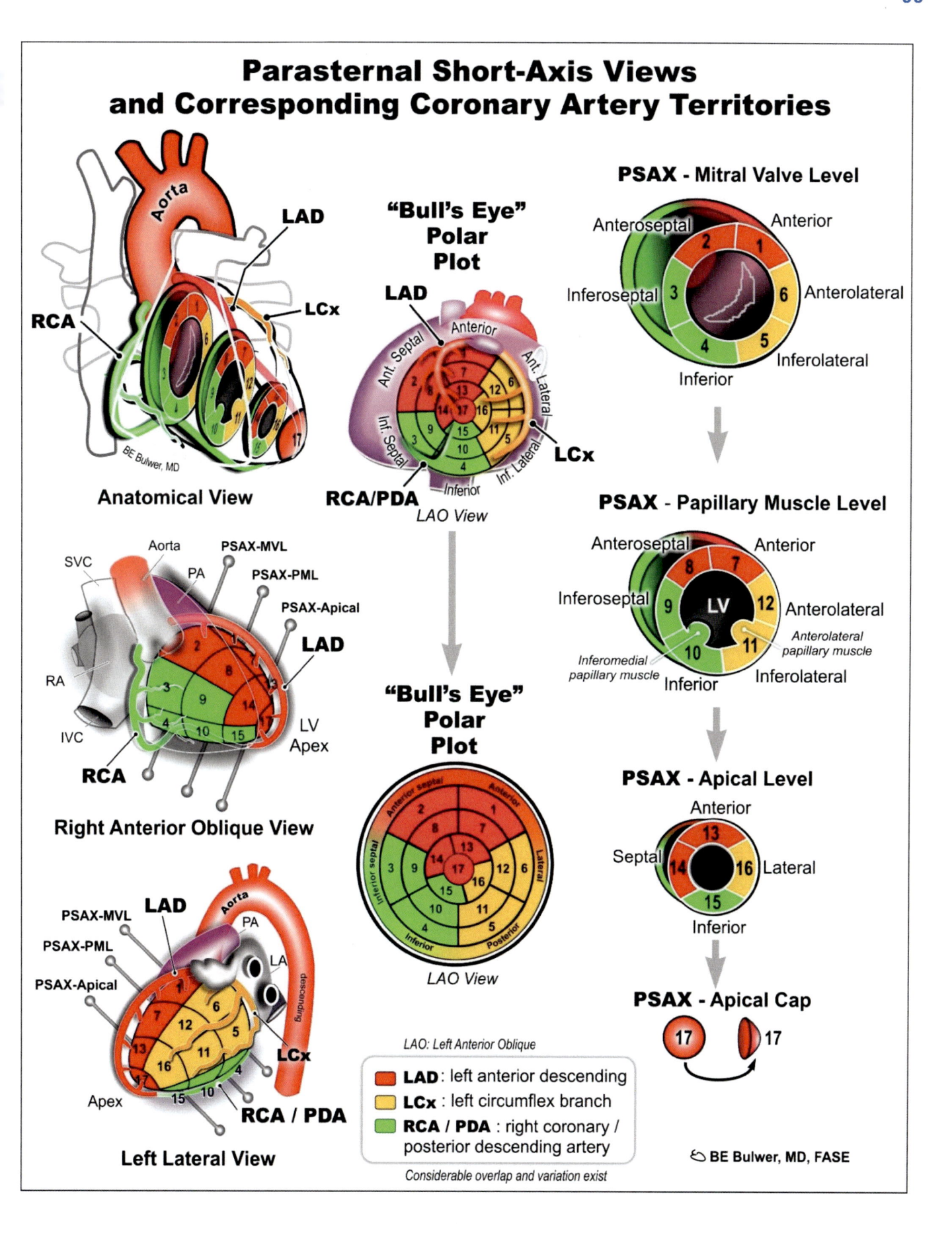

Coronary Artery Territories

Parasternal Short-Axis Views and Corresponding Coronary Artery Territories

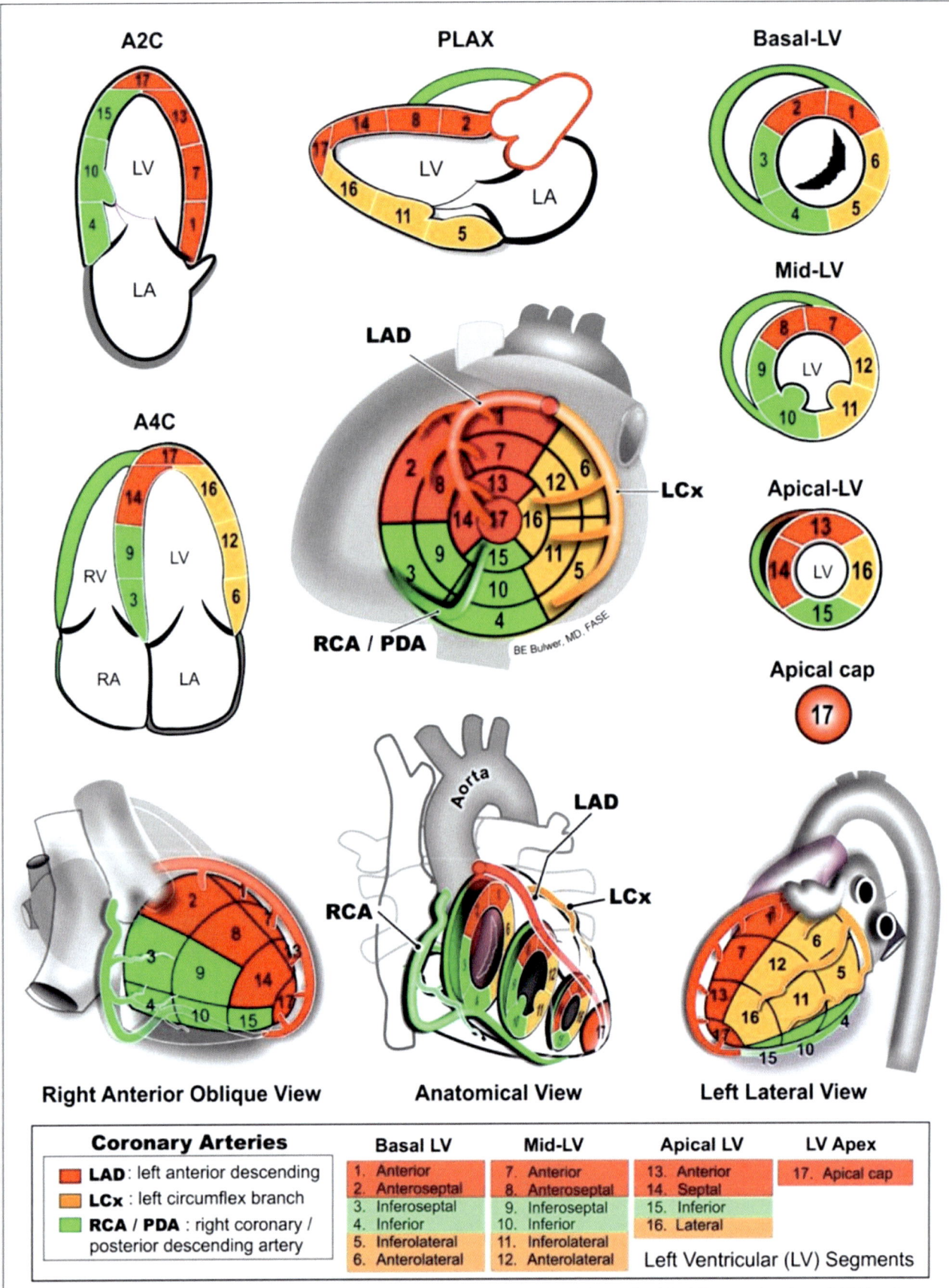

Echocardiography Illustrated

Coronary Artery Territories, Echocardiographic Imaging Planes, and Left Ventricular Segmentation

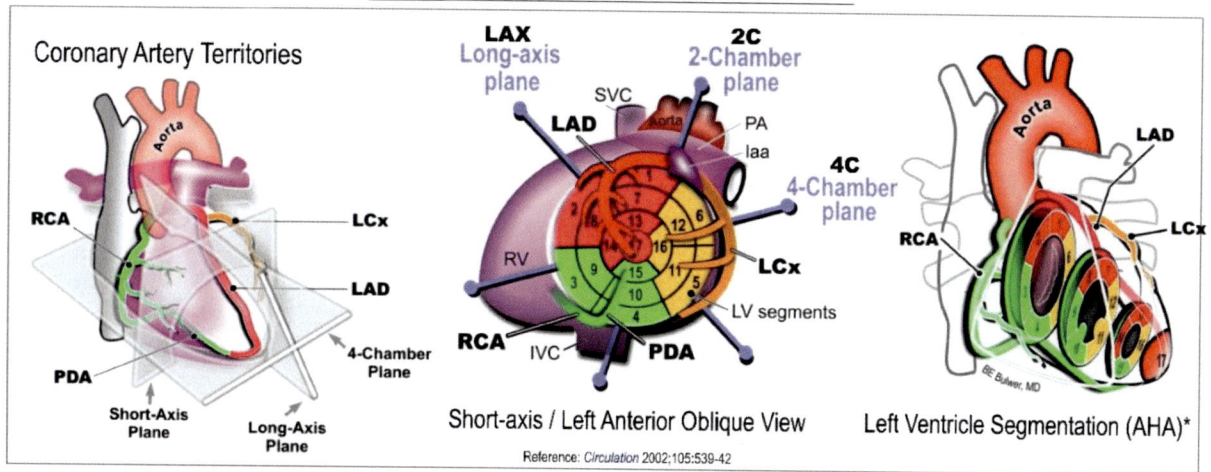

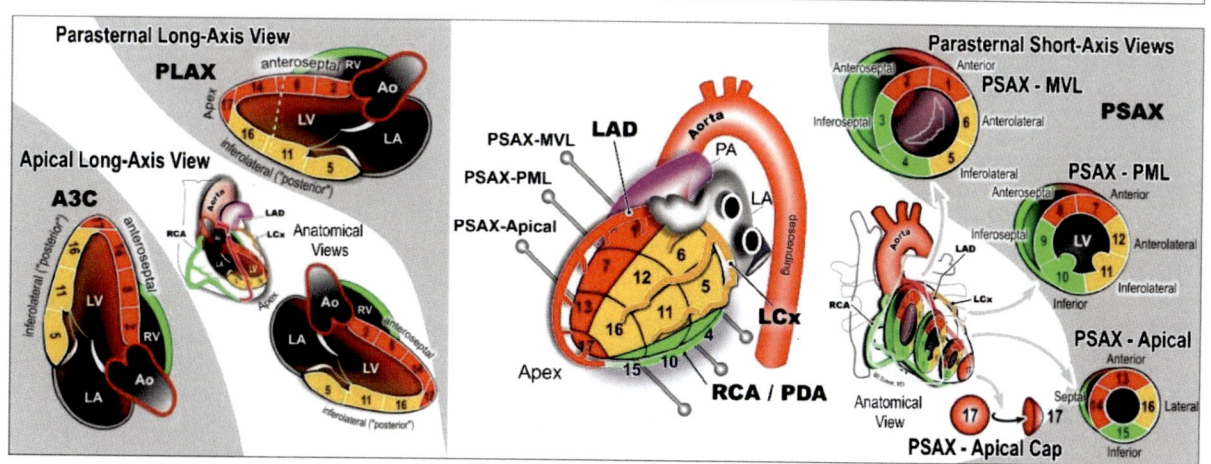

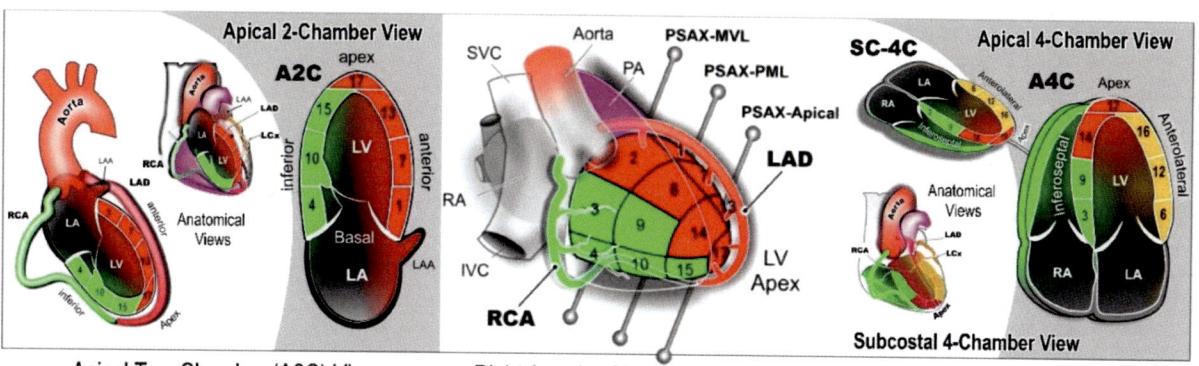

Left Ventricular (LV) Segments

Coronary Arteries	Basal LV	Mid-LV	Apical LV	LV Apex
LAD: left anterior descending	1. basal anterior	7. mid anterior	13. apical anterior	17. apex
LCx: left circumflex branch	2. basal anteroseptal	8. mid anteroseptal	14. apical septal	
RCA / PDA: right coronary / posterior descending artery	3. basal inferoseptal	9. mid inferoseptal	15. apical inferior	
	4. basal inferior	10. mid inferior	16. apical lateral	
	5. basal inferolateral	11. mid inferolateral		
	6. basal anterolateral	12. mid anterolateral		

Considerable overlap and variation exist

Standardized Myocardial Segmentation and Nomenclature. *Circulation* 2002;105:539-42

BE Bulwer, MD, FASE

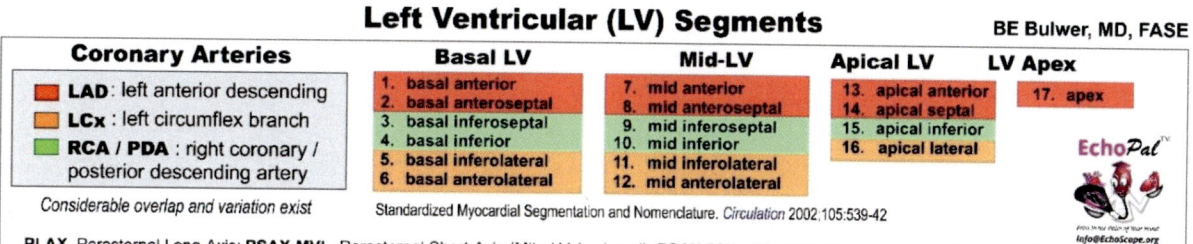

PLAX, Parasternal Long-Axis; **PSAX-MVL**, Parasternal Short-Axis (Mitral Valve Level); **PSAX-PML**, PSAX (Papillary Muscle or Mid-LV Level); **PSAX-Apical**, PSAX (Apical level); **A4C**, Apical 4-Chamber View; **A2C**, Apical 2-Chamber View; **A3C / ALAX**, Apical 3-Chamber or Apical Long-Axis View

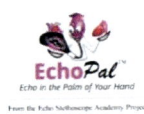

Echocardiography Illustrated Series

	Book Titles: Echocardiography Illustrated Series	Date
	Adult Echo Protocol: English, 2nd ed. *(62 pages)*	2018
	Adult Echo Protocol: Bilingual Simplified Chinese-English, 2nd ed. *(90 pages)*	2018
	Adult Echo Protocol: Bilingual Traditional Chinese-English, 2nd ed. *(90 pages)*	2018
	Adult Echo Protocol: Simplified + Traditional Chinese-English, 2nd ed. *(116 pages)*	2018
	Echo Anatomy, 2nd ed. *(200 pages)* Includes ASE-SCA Transesophageal Echocardiography [TEE] Views side-by-side with corresponding Transthoracic Echocardiographic [TTE] Views);	2018
	Transthoracic Echocardiography: Foundations of Image Acquisition and Interpretation, 3rd ed. *(590 pages)*	2020
	Coronary Artery Territories, 2nd ed. *(110 pages)*	June 2020
	Ventricular Systolic Function, 2nd ed. *(165 pages)*	June 2020
	Ventricular Diastolic Function, 2nd ed. *(65 pages)*	June 2020
	Echo Physiology and Hemodynamics, 2nd ed. *(275 pages)*	June 2020
	How to Do an Echo Exam, 3rd ed. *(590 pages)* *Expanded with: Illustrated Reference Guides include: ASE Chamber Quantification, Transesophageal Echocardiography (TEE) Views (side by side), Introduction to Ultrasound Physics, Instruments and Knobology, Tissue Harmonic Imaging, Contrast-Enhanced Echocardiography, Three-Dimensional (3D) Echocardiography*	April 26, 2020
	Ultrasound Physics: Introduction to Doppler and B-Mode Echocardiography, 1st ed. *(312 pages)*	April 30, 2020
	Ultrasound Physics: B-Mode Echocardiography with introduction to Doppler, 1st ed. *(590 pages)*	March 31, 2020
	Transthoracic Echocardiography: Foundations of Image Acquisition and Interpretation, 3rd ed. *(590 pages)*	April 24, 2020

Contact: *Author@EchoScope.org*

Print and Kindle eBook edition @ Amazon.com

Made in the USA
Middletown, DE
28 December 2024